GERIATRIC
LONG-TERM
PROCEDURES

TREATMENTS

A Problem-Solving Approach

MARIE JAFFE, R.N., M.S.

Skidmore-Roth Publishing, Inc.

PUBLISHING

Jaffe, Marie S.
Geriatric Long-Term Procedures & Treatments/Marie S. Jaffe

ISBN 0-944132-97-9
1. Nursing-Handbooks, Manuals.
2. Medical-Handbooks, Manuals.

SKIDMORE-ROTH PUBLISHING, INC.
7730 Trade Center Avenue
El Paso, TX 79912
1(800)825-3150

TABLE OF CONTENTS

❧

UNIT V.
Medication Administration

UNIT VI.
Intravenous Therapy

UNIT XII.
Musculoskeletal Procedures

UNIT XIII.
Integumentary Procedures

UNIT XIV.
Specimen Procedures

UNIT XV.
Emergency Procedures

UNIT XVI
Psychosocial Procedures

TABLE OF CONTENTS EXPANDED

UNIT III
Vital Signs Procedures

UNIT IV
Personal Hygiene Procedures

UNIT V
Medication Administration Procedures

UNIT IX
Pulmonary Procedures

UNIT X
Renal/Urologic Procedures

UNIT XI
Gastrointestinal Procedures

UNIT XII
Musculoskeletal Procedures

UNIT XIII
Integumentary Procedures

UNIT XIV
Specimen Procedures

UNIT XV
Emergency Procedures

UNIT XVI
Psychosocial Procedures

INTRODUCTION

Geriatric Long-Term Procedures and Treatments focuses on the provision of safe and competent care in long-term, alternative or assistive care facilities while promoting the comfort and privacy needs of the geriatric client/resident. In this respect, it differs from the hospital procedures and care given for more acute conditions. The book is divided into 16 general systems and 124 procedures and treatments related to those systems. In total, 300 specific procedures and treatments are discussed and identified by their own titles or clustered within the associated headings. The degree of difficulty for each procedure differs, ranging from very basic skills to those of greater complexity—skills that can be performed by different levels of personnel, such as, registered nurses (RN), licensed vocational/practical nurses (LVN or LPN), or nursing assistants (NA). Specific procedures and/or treatments can be performed on a single basis or combined with others to provide the necessary nursing care needed by an individual resident. A good example of this is the resident who requires complete care because of severe weakness, disabilities, or an unconscious state. Another example is the resident that is partially or totally independent in self-care activities who requires minimal assistance and fewer procedures. Inherent in each skill is the attention to psychosocial considerations as well as the performance of physical tasks.

The content for each procedure or treatment is divided into sections that are identified with the nursing process; namely, Assessment, Nursing Diagnoses, Goals, Interventions, and Evaluation to facilitate the application of this problem-solving method.

EACH PROCEDURE CONTAINS

- **Definition:** *describes the nature and importance of the procedure*

- **Assessment:** *identifies skill performance*

- **Nursing Diagnoses:** *associated with the skill*

- **Goals:** *achieved by performing the skill based on problem identification and/or individual needs*

- **Interventions:** *describes preparation of the resident and required supplies outlined in step-by-step format*

- **Problem-Solving Actions:** *a list of nursing activities that can or should be carried out and the possible modifications that can enhance the effectiveness of the procedure or treatment*

- **Evaluation:** *general suggestions of outcomes that can be expected in order for the stated goal to be achieved*

A reference at the end of the book will provide some resources used in the development of the book and some additional readings that are useful in the performance of the procedures and treatments in this book.

To the best of my knowledge, the procedure and treatment information is accurate and conforms to the standards of care at the time of publication. The manufacturer's informational brochures or inserts that give directions for using hospital equipment should be followed when available.

My thanks and appreciation to Linda Skidmore-Roth, Brenda Goodner, and their staff for their support in the writing and publication of this book.

Marie S. Jaffe

UNIT I

GENERAL FACILITY PROCEDURES

- Admission/Readmission

- Discharge/Transfer

- Documentation

- Postmortem Management

- Resident Rights

ADMISSION/READMISSION

Admission care facilitates the adaptation of an individual to a facility. It includes procedures that prepare for a short-term or long-term stay following hospitalization. How the individual adapts and responds to a stay in the facility depends upon the sensitivity and concern shown during the admission process. Important parts of the resident's stay include activities to support environmental considerations, admission information, orientation, comfort measures, and the care of personal belongings and valuables. The resident should be introduced to the staff and agency regulations, as well as to the procedures. A smooth admission process can relieve anxiety associated with relocation and promote cooperation needed for effective care.

Readmission care facilitates the return of an individual to the facility following a hospitalization or therapeutic leave. It includes a review of the initial admission activities with reinforcement where needed and an update of information regarding health status.

ASSESSMENT

Reason for admission/readmission, room location, general mental condition, presence of family or legal representative, medical diagnoses and admitting orders, initial history and physical/mental assessment, ability of resident to provide information, level of care needed, need for the coordination of different health care providers, advance directive status

NURSING DIAGNOSES

Anxiety; Relocation Stress Syndrome; Ineffective Individual Coping; Powerlessness

GOALS

Smooth transition to stay in the facility with accommodation to personal needs, all-inclusive admission/readmission procedure

INTERVENTIONS

Equipment/Supplies

- Admission package with items to perform personal hygiene care
- Bedpan and/or urinal
- Water pitcher and glass
- Denture cup if needed
- Stethoscope, sphygmomanometer, and thermometer

- Ophthalmoscope/otoscope, kit for neurologic assessment
- Special equipment or supplies (oxygen, suction, irrigation)
- Container for urine specimen and other specimens needed
- Admitting forms and pen

Resident

- Gown to wear and sheet to drape for physical assessment
- Place in position of comfort for examinations, interview, and observations

❧ PROCEDURE

1. Welcome the individual and introduce yourself and others in the immediate vicinity, especially if there is a roommate; ensure that an identification bracelet is in place and validate the proper spelling of the full name and resident number.

2. Include family members in the introductions and other admission activities.

3. Review the medical diagnoses and physician orders.

4. Inquire about any problems that need immediate attention.

5. Orient the resident to the room environment that includes the bed and operation, lighting, ventilation, call light, intercommunications system, telephone use, bedside/overbed table, drawers/closet space, bathroom, private space for belongings, television and radio, and demonstrate the operation of the equipment.

6. Inform of daily routines for meals, personal care, medications, other treatments and possible schedule changes.

7. Inform of visiting time, private space for visiting; provide written policies regarding services available and payment requirements.

8. List and place personal funds or valuables in a bag, have resident or family member sign, and send to safe, provide safe storage for prostheses and aids if needed (dentures, glasses, hearing aid, artificial eye, or limb).

9. Perform interview for admission history and complete the admission/readmission assessment emphasizing vital signs, specimen collections, baseline for activities of daily living, functional status of each system, skin check for red/open areas, and complaints; perform handwashing prior to hands-on activities.

10. At conclusion of admission care, leave resident in comfortable position dressed in a gown or daytime clothing as desired.

11. Inform the resident and family that questions and concerns are welcomed and will be answered and/or clarified. They should feel free to approach staff for information.

12. Notify the attending physician of the admission; compile a new clinical record and document pertinent admission information.

❧ PROBLEM-SOLVING ACTIONS

1. Repeat information as needed if there are questions; speak clearly and slowly and secure the assistance of an interpreter if needed.

2. Remove medications brought from home. Store the medication or send home with a family member.

3. Advise the resident and visitors of smoking regulations to prevent accidental fire or complaints by other residents.

4. If readmission is anticipated, inform of the bed-holding policy in writing prior to leaving the facility.

❧ EVALUATION

Entry into the facility with anxiety at a manageable level; admission/readmission procedure performed without incident

DISCHARGE/TRANSFER

Discharge care terminates a short-term stay at a facility. It includes the planning and preparation of the resident and family for continuity of physical, emotional, and social care. The discharge plan focuses on the communication of information, instructions for performing procedures and giving care, referrals, and coordination of services. Caregiver assistance and support is also a component of the discharge procedure.

A transfer moves the resident within or outside of the facility. It can be done within the facility if a different unit or room is requested, or if a different level of care is needed. It can be done outside the facility if the needs cannot be met in the facility. In either case, appropriate information and personal belongings should accompany the resident to ensure safe, continuous care.

Discharge or transfer of a resident can be initiated by physician order or by resident and/or family demand. If a change is initiated by the facility, a written notice that includes the reason, date, location and name of destination must be given to the resident and family as required by law.

ASSESSMENT

General mental and physical condition; readiness for discharge; level of care needed; information and instruction needed; need for environmental modification and coordination of different health providers; reason for transfer and name of the new location

NURSING DIAGNOSES

Anxiety; Ineffective Management of Therapeutic Regimen; High Risk for Caregiver Role Strain

GOAL

Discharge or transfer plan formulated and implemented with accommodations for personal considerations and needs

INTERVENTIONS

Equipment/Supplies

- Wheelchair or stretcher
- All personal belongings in a suitcase or bag with the admission list of belongings
- Medications and prescriptions
- Appropriate forms, clinical record for discharge or transfer as applicable

Resident

- Dress in appropriate clothing for discharge or transfer
- Place in position of comfort in the wheelchair or on the stretcher

PROCEDURE

1. Perform handwashing.
2. Provide information and reason for transfer within or outside of facility.

3. Assemble all belongings, supplies, medications, proper forms and records, including an assessment and plan summary to accompany the transfer of a resident to another facility or acute care center.

4. Complete all teaching involving diet, activities, medications, treatments, physician appointments, complaints to report; provide instructions in written form to reinforce teaching.

5. Formulate a plan of maintenance care with other interdisciplinary members in writing and give to the resident and family; include self-care options.

6. Assemble all personal belongings and valuables, check against admission list and pack or place in a bag.

7. Provide referral information and assist with coordination of resources and providers of care (physical, mental, social, emotional, legal, financial).

8. Document discharge or transfer plan and other pertinent information in the clinical record.

9. Provide for appropriate transportation if needed.

10. Perform room check to ensure that all belongings are removed and accompany the resident when discharged or transferred.

❧ PROBLEM-SOLVING ACTIONS

1. Notify the appropriate departments of the discharge or transfer.

2. Provide telephone numbers to resident, family, and facility for use if additional information is needed.

3. Involve the family in all planning, preparation, and instruction.

4. Special care should be given to those discharged or transferred with a dressing, catheters, or those who need continuous treatment, such as oxygen.

❧ EVALUATION

Discharge or transfer procedure performed smoothly and comprehensively

DOCUMENTATION

Documentation is the recording of all information, both objective and subjective, in the clinical record of an individual resident. It includes observations, investigations, and communications of the resident involving care and treatments. It has legal requirements regarding accuracy and completeness, legibility and timing. Special forms in the clinical record are utilized in nursing documentation, such as, assessment, care plan, nursing progress notes, flow sheets, medication sheets, incident reports, and summary sheets (daily, weekly, monthly, and discharge). All documentation and clinical records are confidential and can be released only with signed permission of the resident.

ASSESSMENT

Clinical record that contains all necessary forms and blank sheets identified with the resident's name, physician's name, room and resident numbers

NURSING DIAGNOSES

None

GOAL

Complete, accurate, accessible documentation on the appropriate sheet in the clinical record

INTERVENTIONS

Equipment/Supplies

- Complete systematically organized clinical record in a protective cover
- Ball point pen, black ink

Resident

- None

PROCEDURES

1. Include family or legal representative information in front of clinical record.
2. Place nursing alert stickers such as allergies on the front cover of the record.
3. Place all required and appropriately signed forms in the clinical record, such as, "advance directive," permissions for specific procedures, consult results, laboratory, diagnostic procedure, history and physical reports, others as applicable.
4. Review documents to determine need for follow-up monitoring, and laboratory tests and procedures. Ensure that active diagnoses are transferred from hospital forms to the appropriate facility forms.
5. Document identifying and statistical information on the proper sheet.
6. Document completed assessments in a timely manner:
   a. Admission assessment
   b. Comprehensive assessment
   c. Quarterly, annual, and periodic assessments (daily for unstable systems)
7. Document a comprehensive care plan:
   a. Immediate care plan for acute conditions
   b. Nursing diagnoses

   c. Goals to be achieved

   d. Interventions and services including interdisciplinary activities

   e. Evaluations of goals and actions taken to solve the problem

   f. Revisions of the care plan when appropriate

8. Complete documentation in narrative nursing notes in a timely manner:
   a. Daily documentation for each shift on new admissions, during and following an acute episode, following an incident, and during physiologic, mental or emotional changes or instability
   b. Weekly summary documentation on those requiring acute care
   c. Monthly or biweekly documentation on those requiring unskilled care

9. Document or check information on flow sheets each shift or as appropriate for the care or treatment being monitored.

10. Use only accepted and approved abbreviations in documentation.

11. Include initials or proper signature on all entries; cosign documentation of other staff members when necessary or according to policy.

12. Comply with all legal requirements of documentation:
    a. Use pen for notations.
    b. Write neatly and legibly.
    c. Do not erase, correct mistakes by drawing a line through the content to be deleted and initial.
    d. Maintain cleanliness of the record, avoid spills or other accidents that will obliterate the writing.
    e. Never use liquid paper or in any way cover documentation.
    f. Never throw away any page from the document.

13. Retain and protect documentation in the clinical record from loss, destruction, or unauthorized use; maintain confidentiality of documentation and other contents of the clinical record and release information only with permission of the resident or if required by law or insurance contract.

❧ PROBLEM SOLVING ACTIONS

1. Documentation can include the nursing diagnosis and goal identification.

2. Flow sheets are often used for activities and procedures that are performed frequently.

3. If computerized documentation is used, safeguards and controls to protect data from changes should be present; each authorized person must have a personal identifier and electronic signature based on qualifications to access and enter data.

❧ EVALUATION

Completed and accurate documentation on all appropriate clinical record sheets, information is comprehensive and timely and properly signed

POSTMORTEM MANAGEMENT

Postmortem management includes a combination of physical care, preparation of the body for viewing by the family, transportation to the funeral home, care of all personal belongings, and appropriate legal notification and documentation. It also includes support of the family members during this time of grief, and consideration for religious beliefs and spiritual needs. Agency policies should be followed in addition to or in place of the suggested care outlined in this procedure.

ASSESSMENT

Time that death is pronounced, family members present and request to view the body, religious affiliation and beliefs about care after death, funeral or other arrangements and special permits, if needed

NURSING DIAGNOSES

Altered Family Processes; Anticipatory or Actual Grieving; Ineffective Family Coping: Compromised

GOAL

Dignified care of the deceased resident and family members

INTERVENTIONS

Equipment/Supplies

- Basin or warm water, soap, wash cloth, and towel
- Disposable gloves
- Clean gown or shroud
- Clean linens as needed
- Dressings, absorbent pads, gauze rolls, cottonballs, and tape
- Bags for personal belongings and list of valuables
- Identification tags (3)

Resident

- Place in supine position in proper body alignment with head slightly elevated on a small pillow
- Raise bed to working level

PROCEDURE

1. Perform handwashing.
2. Become familiar with assessment data and agency policies regarding postmortem management, family request to view body.
3. Confirm death pronouncement by physician or according to policy.
4. Notify departments, official agencies, personnel, funeral home, and clergy as needed or requested.
5. Provide privacy while performing care.
6. Remove soiled gown, tubes, equipment, dressings.
7. Elevate the head of the bed to prevent pooling of blood or fluid to the head that will cause discoloration, gently close the eyes, and place dentures in the mouth.

8. Cleanse the body and dry thoroughly, redress any open or draining wounds, groom hair, and change any linens needed if the family wishes to view the body.

9. Place absorbent pads under the buttocks and between the legs.

10. Stabilize chin with a small rolled towel to close mouth if needed.

11. Provide a clean gown or shroud.

12. If body is to be viewed by family members:
    a. Remove all equipment and supplies and put the room in order.
    b. Cover body with a clean sheet to shoulder level.
    c. Provide privacy or stay with family and give comfort and support if family requests this.

13. Following the viewing of the body by the family, loosely tie the ankles and wrist with roller gauze, support chin with chin straps tied on top to the head, place pads on eyes and secure with a bandage; use padding under all ties to prevent bruising or damage as the cooling process causes loss of skin elasticity and any trauma or pressure can result in discoloration or tears.

14. Prepare three identification tags with the resident's name, physician's name, facility name and room number; allow wrist band to remain to serve as further identification.

15. Secure an identification tag on the resident's great toe, wrist, or ankle and wrap body in a sheet or shroud and secure a second identification tag to the covering.

16. Assemble all belongings and valuables and place in a bag and attach the third identification tag, double check belongings and have family sign for them when received.

17. Take the body to the morgue or allow to remain in the room until the funeral home comes for it according to agency policy; have funeral director sign receipt for body.

18. Complete all forms and records.

☙ PROBLEM-SOLVING ACTIONS

1. Carry out same protective procedures implemented by staff if the resident received isolation precautions (gown, gloves, linen, body fluids, environment, others as applicable). A written explanation about the type of protective care needed should accompany the body.

2. Discuss and clarify questions about organ donations if applicable.

3. Provide explanations if death is to be reported to an official agency, this procedure is done if death occurred under unusual circumstances.

4. Have a witness verify belongings and valuables before bagging and giving them to the family.

5. Include any money maintained by the agent for the resident's expenses in the belongings returned to the family.

6. Some residents have a legal representative to handle all decisions and finances; this person can replace a family for funeral and other arrangements.

7. Postmortem care should be completed as soon after death as possible as rigor mortis begins in 2 to 4 hours causing stiffness from muscle contraction and immobilization of the joints.

☙ EVALUATION

Complete the appropriate care given to the deceased; family support facilitated and needs fulfilled

RESIDENT RIGHTS

Resident rights provide and ensure the promotion and protection of dignity and confidentiality, self-determination, and communication. They include freedom of choice in care and treatments, activities and participation, physician and dentist or other professionals, freedom from abuse or discrimination, and protection in healthcare in the form of an "advance directive." The "advance directive" is a legal document that contains written instructions regarding healthcare, treatments, and procedures to be accepted or rejected in the event of incompetency. The directive can name a legal representative to act on behalf of a resident if this becomes necessary. All notices of rights and responsibilities and policy changes regarding these rights must be given in writing and communicated orally to residents.

ASSESSMENT

Notification of rights, competency and ability and interest in making choices and exercising rights, complaints from residents or family members regarding rights violation

NURSING DIAGNOSES

Anxiety; Self-Esteem Disturbance; Decisional Conflict (Treatments and Care to Accept or Reject)

GOAL

Protection and promotion of resident rights

PROCEDURES

1. Provide resident with "Resident's Bill of Rights," Standards of Gerontological Nursing Practice. Facility rules, regulations, and policies in writing and discuss and clarify in understandable language.

2. Provide information about "advance directive" and assist in complying with this right based on the resident's choice, document that this information has been provided:
   a. Living Will
   b. Medical Durable Power of Attorney
   c. Legal representative
   d. Include refusal or acceptance of any medical or surgical procedure or care
   e. Place copy in the clinical record
   f. Honor all stated desires in the document including "Do Not Resuscitate" orders

3. Provide privacy and confidentiality in personal care, treatments, clinical records, and communications.

4. Allow for choice of physician, dentist, other professionals as needed.

5. Allow for individual religious affiliation and participation if desired.

6. Include in care planning choices, schedules, and participation in activities.

7. Protect personal funds and belongings from theft or loss by placing them in the safe.

8. Provide a safe environment and private space for visits from family, friends, and health care professionals.

9. Provide and assist with telephone and mail services and ensure privacy.

10. Provide for absentee voting and other rights of citizenship.

11. Allow for refusal of treatment or care and avoid reprisal or coercion of choices made by the resident in exercising rights.

❧ PROBLEM-SOLVING ACTIONS

1. Assess and provide for grievance procedure and give assistance when needed.
2. Provide self-administration of medication if able to manage this safely.
3. Record mental changes observed that can affect ability to make own choices and exercise rights.
4. Ensure that staff members and others involved in care know about wishes and requests made by the resident.
5. Act as an advocate on behalf of the resident in situations involving unsafe or inadequate care, discrimination or abuse, and report to the proper authorities for resolution.
6. Investigate state law regarding "advance directive" to ensure legality of the document.

❧ EVALUATION

Resident choices and rights promoted and protected in all areas with encouragement to participate in decision-making

UNIT II

INFECTION CONTROL PROCEDURES

- Handwashing Technique
- Isolation Management
- Sterile/Clean Technique
- Universal Precautions

HANDWASHING TECHNIQUE

Handwashing is performed by personnel to remove microorganisms and contaminants from the hands and nails. It is done to prevent transmission of transient bacteria to the resident receiving care. It requires the use of soap or other agents, a source of running water, and the friction of rubbing the hands together. It is recommended that the procedure be performed before and after every contact with a resident and after the handling or touching of contaminated articles or equipment, before and after eating, after using the bathroom, when manipulating contact lenses, and any other activities involving body secretions.

ASSESSMENT

Determination of clean or contaminated activity, condition of the skin of personnel's hands (dry, cracks, lesions, rash, hangnails)

NURSING DIAGNOSES

High Risk for Infection; High Risk for Impaired Skin Integrity (Personnel)

GOALS

Transmission of pathogens to susceptible resident minimized; intact skin on hands of personnel; correct performance of handwashing based on assessment data

INTERVENTIONS

Equipment/Supplies

- Soap from dispenser, antiseptic soap or foam
- Running water with ability to adjust temperature
- Paper towels in dispenser

- Disposable gloves
- Nail file or orangewood cuticle stick
- Waste receptacle

Resident

- Explain purpose of handwashing and importance of washing own hands before and after certain activities
- Access to water, soap, and towels within reach

PROCEDURE

1. Remove rings, except for smooth-finished wedding band, and place watch above wrist on forearm as these articles harbor and promote growth of microorganisms.

2. Adjust temperature to a warm, comfortable level with a moderate flow to prevent splashing and to promote removal of microorganisms.

3. Wet hands under the running water while holding them downward to allow the water to run from arm to fingertips to the sink (cleanest to dirtiest areas.)

4. Obtain soap from the dispenser and lather between both hands.

5. To produce friction, rub hands together in a circular motion and wash each finger separately.

6. Include wrist area and nail beds by massaging; use orangewood stick if needed.

7. Washing procedure should take from 10 seconds to 2 minutes depending on whether clean or sterile technique is required.

8. Rinse each hand thoroughly under running water with fingers pointed downward; avoid touching sink as it is considered a contaminated area.

9. Repeat the procedure a second time if hands or activity has been determined to be contaminated or according to guidelines for universal precautions.

10. Dry hands, one at a time, with paper towels and patting motion.

11. Turn off faucet with paper towel and discard in wastebasket to prevent contamination.

PROBLEM-SOLVING ACTIONS

1. Use cleansing agents based on whether activity is determined to be clean or contaminated; the antiseptic agents should be reserved for more contaminated activities where the risk of infection is high, or where water is not available.

2. The length of time required for handwashing is determined according to the type of activity (clean or contaminated); generally, 10 seconds to 2 minutes is sufficient.

3. Handwashing may be reduced if tasks are performed from the cleanest to the dirtiest areas.

4. Lotions and hand creams should not be used after handwashing as they are not sterile and are a source of pathogenic microorganisms.

5. Personnel's skin problems of the hands should be treated and gloves should be worn while giving care; rough or torn nails, hangnails, or chipped polish on nails should be avoided and given proper attention.

EVALUATION

Properly performed handwashing procedure for appropriate length of time and at appropriate times based on assessment, hands of personnel intact and considered free of contaminants

ISOLATION MANAGEMENT

Isolation management is a method of infection control requiring specific practices based on the type of isolation to be implemented. These are outlined in guidelines developed by the Centers for Disease Control (CDC) for disease categories (respiratory) or disease specific (abscess). The most common isolation system used is the category specific and includes strict isolation, contact isolation, respiratory isolation, enteric precautions, and blood/body fluid/drainage/secretion/excretion precautions. Protective, or reverse, isolation is not an official CDC category. Some physicians may order it when a resident is extremely immunosuppressed. All levels require labeling and bagging of contaminated materials.

ASSESSMENT

Disease or disorder and identified pathogenic microorganism, physical and emotional status, identified type and level of isolation precautions needed, use of equipment that has a potential for harboring pathogens

NURSING DIAGNOSES

High Risk for Infection; Impaired Social Interaction; Ineffective Individual Coping

GOALS

Minimal transmission potential of pathogens to or from resident; effective measures implemented to protect resident and/or staff from pathogens

INTERVENTIONS

Equipment/Supplies

- Private room if on strict or protective isolation
- Disposable gowns, masks, and other protective clothing and items on a cart inside or outside the room
- Disposable packaged supplies and equipment (needles, syringes, dressings, linens, tissues, others as needed)
- Separate laundry hamper
- Wastebasket with plastic liner

- Isolation bags of various sizes, colors and tags
- Biohazard container

- Disinfectant solution and detergent

- Handwashing utensils and liquid antiseptic soap

Resident

- Explain purpose, type of isolation and expected results

PROCEDURE

1. Provide a private room or allocate the amount of space needed between residents as recommended by the CDC guidelines to establish a physical barrier; move a resident if the roommate is a high risk for infection.

2. Perform handwashing before and after each contact with resident whether gloves are worn or not, and following exposure to any contaminant (see Handwashing Technique).

3. Wear disposable gloves to protect hands from possible contact with body fluid or contaminated article, to draw blood or administer parenteral medications or fluids, or to collect or handle specimens.

4. Provide protective clothing based on the type of isolation:
   a. Disposable gown application and removal:
      - Pick up the gown and unfold while holding at the top.
      - Hold the gown with the opening toward your body and slip the arms into the sleeves.
      - Adjust the gown by overlapping the two sides at the back and tie; tie at the neck if strings are present.
      - To remove, untie strings at neck and back and pull off shoulders and sleeves turning the gown inside out while the gloves remain on the hands.
      - Fold or roll gown while it is inside out and discard it into the lined wastebasket, avoid touching the outside of the gown.
      - Remove gloves as outlined in "c" below.
   b. Mask application and removal:
      - Adjust mask over nose and mouth.
      - Place and adjust elastic band or tie around head to secure the mask.
      - Gently press the small metal band over the top of the nose.
      - Remove by pulling elastic over the head and the mask from the nose and mouth and discard in the plastic-lined wastebasket.
      - Avoid touching the outside of the mask.
   c. Disposable gloves application and removal:
      - Grasp the cuff of the glove and slip on the hand with one smooth movement; if gown is worn, pull the top of the glove over the gown sleeves.
      - Remove the first glove by grasping the cuffs and pulling downward turning the glove inside out and discard in the lined wastebasket.

5. Dispose of items based on type of item:
   a. Disposable items such as tubes, containers, dressings, protective clothing, dishes and utensils, gloves, linens, and any other contaminated articles:
      - Double bag and apply biohazard label.
      - Place used needles and syringes in a biohazard container without replacing the cap over the needle or removing or bending the needle; avoid any needle sticks when placing the articles in the container.
   b. Reusable items such as dishes, linens, equipment used for treatments, and other articles used:
      - Wash dishes in dishwasher and allow to hot dry.
      - Double bag linen and secure with ties, and label according to facility policy.
      - Wash equipment and soak in a germicidal solution, rinse well and dry.

6. Dispose of urine, feces, and drainage using gloves based on type of isolation and reason for special handling.

7. Collect and handle specimens using gloves, applying a lid, label and bag for transport to the laboratory.

8. Perform and maintain activities outlined for the type of isolation precautions to be implemented:
   a. Strict isolation: gown, gloves, mask, private room, disposable dishes; all items in room are considered contaminated
   b. Contact isolation: gown, gloves, mask, private room, gloves for anyone in contact with patient; all articles in contact with patient considered contaminated

   NOTE: The primary difference between strict isolation and contact isolation is that strict isolation prevents the transmission of highly contagious infections that can be spread by both air and contact; contact isolation prevents the spread of highly transmissible infections that are generally spread by close or direct contact.

   c. Respiratory isolation: mask, gown, gloves
   d. Enteric isolation: gown, gloves
   e. Wound/skin precautions: gown, gloves, mask
   f. Blood/body fluids/secretions/excretion precautions: gown, gloves

❧ PROBLEM-SOLVING ACTIONS

1. Screen visitors and staff for illness or infections; limit number of visitors if necessary; avoid scheduling staff who are ill.

2. Instruct and assist visitors to perform isolation precautions and handwashing.

3. Replace gown, mask, glove supply as needed as well as items needed for care and treatments; never reuse any item that has not been cleaned after use.

4. Notify other departments involved in care or procedures of the isolation precautions.

❧ EVALUATION

Correct performance of procedures to maintain an identified level of isolation; no evidence of spread of pathogens to the resident or others

STERILE/CLEAN TECHNIQUE

Sterile technique is a method of maintaining the sterility of all articles and establishing barriers to maintain a sterile field. It is used in the delivery of care or treatments involving a break or potential for a break in the body's defenses, as well as sterile body cavities. Some of these procedures include wound dressing and care, care of any tubes and insertion sites, and care of areas that are potential sites of contamination. Sterile technique requires that everything involved in a procedure be sterile and remain sterile from initiation to completion.

Clean technique (sometimes called "no-touch technique") is a method of performing care and treatments using sterile articles without touching or contaminating the part of the sterile item that will be exposed to the area to be treated. This method is used for simple dry dressing changes and other procedures that can be performed without a sterile field or sterile gloves but still need a level of medical asepsis to prevent complications.

ASSESSMENT

Body part and type of care to be given, physical and mental status and need for protection, medical diagnoses

NURSING DIAGNOSES

High Risk for Infection; Impaired Skin Integrity

GOALS

Maintenance of sterile or clean technique in performance of procedures, correct use and care of sterile supplies in the performance of sterile or clean technique

INTERVENTIONS

Equipment/Supplies

- Sterile gloves of correct size
- Sterile packaged dressings
- Sterile forceps
- Sterile packaged antiseptic swabs
- Sterile packaged towels
- Sterile solutions and containers
- Sterile tubes or other packaged articles
- Other packaged sterile items as needed
- Sterile lubricants or ointments
- Tape

Resident

- Explain purpose and type of procedure
- Place in a position that allows for access to the treatment area

PROCEDURE

1. Perform handwashing before and after each procedure whether or not sterile gloves are worn (see Handwashing Technique); a 2-minute handwashing is advised for sterile and clean technique procedures.
2. Assemble the sterile supplies needed for the specific procedure.
3. Set up the sterile field as follows:
   a. Prepare a clean dry surface within reach of the working area.

b. Open sterile packages of towels correctly and pick up by the corners, allow to unfold, and place it on the surface moving it from the farthest to nearest areas while avoiding contamination of the area that is to remain sterile.

4. Open sterile packages needed and place items on the sterile field:
    a. Open heat sealed packages by grasping the top flaps and pulling apart, hold over the field and carefully place onto the sterile surface.
    b. Open heat sealed packages by grasping the top flaps and pulling apart completely; lay it on a flat surface with sterile contents exposed if clean technique is to be performed.
    c. Open wrapped cloth by laying the cloth flat on a surface or by holding it with the nondominant hand; open the farthest top flap, reach around and open the right and left flap with the respective hands if lying flat or with the dominant hand being held, then open the front flap by moving it forward.
    d. If the item is to be added to the field, grasp the ends under the package with the dominant hand and hold in place while dropping the sterile contents onto the field without allowing any contact with an unsterile area.
    e. Arrange items on the field with the sterile forceps removed from its package and rest the forceps with the sterile part on the field and the handles outside or on the edge of the field; or open and place the sterile forceps on the field.
    f. Dispose of paper or cloth covers appropriately.

5. Pour sterile solution into a container either on or off a sterile field:
    a. Check label on the bottle to ensure that the correct solution is poured; check container for evidence of contamination.
    b. Remove bottle top or seal and place on a surface with the open side up.
    c. Avoid touching the top, seal, rim or inside of the bottle.
    d. Move the container as near to the edge as possible with the forceps or a nondominant, sterile gloved hand.
    e. Hold bottle firmly with label away from the pouring side and carefully pour the appropriate amount of solution without splashing.
    f. Replace the bottle top and date if solution is to be used again within 24 hours; dispose of bottle if empty.

6. Prepare and put on sterile gloves:
    a. Open the glove package on a flat surface and expose the gloves without touching the inside of the package or the gloves.
    b. Pick up the gloves by the cuff with the nondominant hand and lift it from the wrapper above waist level and away from any possible contamination.
    c. Slip the glove on the dominant hand with fingers properly placed in it and pull over the hand while still touching the inside of the cuff.
    d. With the gloved hand, pick up the remaining glove by slipping the fingers under the cuff.
    e. Slip the second glove on the hand with the fingers properly placed in it; adjust the fingers in the gloves if needed with the other gloved hand.
    f. Maintain the gloved hands above waist level and keep hands in sight to prevent possible contamination.
    g. Remove gloves at the completion of the procedure by pulling one off, holding the inside of the cuff and turning inside out; remove and pull off the second glove by inserting the ungloved fingers inside the glove and turning inside out; gloves are then discarded appropriately.

7. At the completion of a sterile procedure, all used articles and supplies are discarded appropriately according to Universal Precautions and facility policy.

8. To perform clean technique using sterile articles:
    a. Perform handwashing for 2 minutes.
    b. Open all sterile articles as outlined.
    c. Touch only those areas of the sterile item that will not be in contact with the area being treated.

9. To perform clean technique using clean articles:
    a. Perform handwashing for at least 10 seconds.
    b. Ensure that the articles have been washed, rinsed, and disinfected when indicated and allowed to air dry.

c. Avoid allowing clean equipment or supplies to touch unclean areas or allowing hands to touch areas that have direct entrance or exposure to an area being treated, such as, feeding tubes, urinary or fecal diversion tubes, respiratory tubes and inhalation therapy, irrigation.

PROBLEM-SOLVING ACTIONS

1. Validate expiration dates on sterile supplies and equipment.
2. Always check for tears, breaks, or any other indications of contamination of sterile items before using.
3. Be alert for any contamination of sterile items and replace when contamination is suspected.
4. Disposable packaged sterile items should be discarded after use.

EVALUATION

Absence of infection or other complications as a result of a break in sterile or clean technique; appropriate technique used correctly and for the proper procedure

UNIVERSAL PRECAUTIONS

Universal Precautions are those practices performed to prevent and control the transmission of blood-borne pathogens. Universal Precautions apply to tissues, blood, and other body fluids containing blood. All residents are approached as if they are HIV or HBV positive. Procedures include proper handwashing and techniques such as protective clothing (masks, gloves, gowns, face shields, eye goggles) and methods of disposing contaminated articles (linens, blood and body fluids, disposable equipment and supplies, reusable equipment and supplies) and the collection and handling of specimens. Recommended guidelines for Universal Precautions are developed by the Centers for Disease Control (CDC) and required by the Occupational Safety and Health Administration (OSHA). The practices are followed by facilities and their staffs to prevent the transmission of organisms between people and between the environment and people.

ASSESSMENT

Presence of infection or susceptibility to infection, potential hazards for infectious process in individuals or environment, need for isolation and level of management

NURSING DIAGNOSIS

High Risk for Infection

GOALS

Transmission of pathogens from individuals or environment prevented or controlled; correct techniques and procedures; measures taken to minimize spread of microorganisms

INTERVENTIONS

Equipment/Supplies

- Fluid resistant protective clothing (gown, mask, gloves, eye goggles)
- Disposable items needed for care
- Biohazard container
- Laundry bags for contaminated linen
- Bags and labels for used contaminated articles

- Disinfectant solution to clean reusable items and spills; germicidal detergents for laundry
- Handwashing supplies that include an antiseptic liquid soap
- Paper towels, tissues
- Specimen containers and labels if needed

Resident

- Explain purpose of special precautionary measures

PROCEDURE

1. Perform handwashing before and after each contact with resident whether gloves are worn or not and following exposure of hands to body fluids, blood, excretions, or other contaminants (see Handwashing Technique).

2. Wear disposable gloves to protect hands from possible contact with any body fluid or any article contaminated with body fluid, to draw blood or administer parenteral medications or fluids; take measures to prevent needle sticks.

3. Wear protective clothing or devices when administering care:
   a. Disposable gown: If soiling or spattering by body fluids is possible during care and if changing linens or dressings
   b. Mask: If transmission of pathogens is possible during coughing or during suctioning
   c. Eye goggles or face shield: If spattering of body fluids is possible

4. Appropriately care for reusable equipment and supplies:
   a. Double bag used linen with the assistance of another staff member and label appropriately; linen should be laundered with germicidal detergent.
   b. Wash dishes in a dishwasher or with hot water and detergent following a rinsing and soaking in a disinfectant solution.
   c. Remove equipment or parts of equipment, place in a bag and label "to be cleaned and sterilized" before reusing.

5. Appropriately care for disposable equipment and supplies:
   a. Contaminated articles such as dressings, gloves, used tissues, dishes and eating utensils, linens, and any others should be bagged, labeled, and discarded according to facility policies.
   b. Needles and syringes should be disposed of in biohazard puncture-resistant containers intact without their needle covers to prevent sticks and possible transmission of pathogens.

6. Urine and feces should be flushed down the toilet, urinals and bedpans should be cleaned, disinfected, rinsed, and dried according to facility policy.

7. Spills are wiped up with paper towels, the area washed, rinsed and disinfected with a germicidal solution and allowed to dry; gloves should be worn to clean any body fluid spills from any surface; all articles used in the clean up of spills should be bagged, labeled, and incinerated.

8. Perform specimen collections by wearing gloves and avoiding any contact with the material to be tested; container should be covered securely, labeled and placed in a bag to be transported to the laboratory.

9. Perform procedures using aseptic technique when needed and using Universal Precautions for disposal of the used supplies.

❧ PROBLEM-SOLVING ACTIONS

1. Visitors should be made aware of safe practices when in contact with the resident such as handwashing, protective clothing, touching used items.

2. Store the articles needed to perform precautionary procedures in the room or where readily available.

❧ EVALUATION

Proper precaution procedures performed based on accepted guidelines outlined by the CDC. Universal Precautions do not eliminate the need for other category-specific or disease-specific isolation, such as enteric precautions for infectious diarrhea.

UNIT III

VITAL SIGNS

- Blood Pressure, Brachial

- Blood Pressure, Standing/Sitting

- Height and Weight, Standing/Bed/Chair

- Pulse, Apical

- Pulse, Apical/Radial

- Pulse, Peripheral

- Pulse, Radial

- Respirations

- Temperature, Oral/Axillary/Rectal/Aural with Electronic Thermometer

- Temperature, Oral/Axillary/Rectal with Mercury Thermometer

BLOOD PRESSURE, BRACHIAL

*T*he *blood pressure (BP) is the pressure of the blood exerted on the arterial wall of the blood vessels, maintained primarily by left ventricle contraction. The blood pressure is monitored routinely to determine baselines and changes in systolic and diastolic levels associated with medical conditions, especially those related to cardiovascular status. The normal limits are 100-140 for systolic and 50-90 for diastolic. The systolic pressure is the measurement of the maximal pressure exerted against the arterial walls (the first sound heard). The diastolic pressure is the measurement of the minimal pressure exerted against the arterial walls (the last sound heard). Systolic pressure represents the ventricular contraction and diastolic pressure represents the ventricular relaxation; the pulse pressure is the difference between the systolic reading and the diastolic reading. Both are measured in millimeters of mercury (mm Hg) using a mercury sphygmomanometer or by observation of a calibrated dial using an aneroid sphygmomanometer. The brachial blood pressure is usually taken with respirations, pulse, and temperature. The popliteal site may be used if the arms are not available for blood pressure measurement.*

❧ ASSESSMENT

Blood pressure range, increases or decreases from baseline parameters; presence of cardiovascular, renal or other disorders affecting blood pressure; administration of antihypertensive medications

❧ NURSING DIAGNOSES

Decreased Cardiac Output; Fluid Volume Deficit

❧ GOALS

Blood pressure measurement within established baseline parameters; correct monitoring of brachial blood pressure and effect on health status

❧ INTERVENTIONS

Equipment/Supplies

- Mercury or aneroid sphygmomanometer with appropriate size cuff
- Antiseptic sponge
- Stethoscope

Resident

- Explain purpose of procedure and expected results
- Place in position of rest and comfort, supine or sitting for brachial with arm and antecubital space exposed; prone for popliteal with thigh and back of knee exposed

❧ PROCEDURE

1. Perform handwashing.

2. Become familiar with baseline blood pressure readings to serve as a comparison, antihypertensive medications ordered and effectiveness.

3. Inspect and test the equipment for leaks in the cuff, tubing, bulb and connections.

4. Eliminate noises that may interfere with the sounds heard through the stethoscope.

5. Measure arm circumference and use appropriate cuff size (width should be at least 40% and length at least 80% of circumference) as cuffs that are too narrow result in false high readings.

6. Allow resident to rest for 5 minutes before starting the procedure.

7. Check that arm placement is at level of the heart as arm above level results in false low readings, and arm below level results in false high readings.

8. Apply cuff smoothly and snugly over upper arm with tubing centered at antecubital space and edge of cuff 1 inch (2.54 cm) above antecubital space or site at which the brachial pulse is palpated; secure in place with hook or velcro.

9. Place mercury sphygmomanometer on stable, level surface with meniscus at eye level or clip aneroid sphygmomanometer to cuff directly in line of vision.

10. Cleanse ear tips of stethoscope and place in ears, diaphragm of the stethoscope may also be cleansed with antiseptic sponge.

11. Palpate the brachial artery with pads of fingers of the nondominant hand and inflate the cuff with dominant hand until pulsation disappears plus an additional 20 to 30 mm Hg to use as a gauge to ensure cuff is inflated enough to measure systolic pressure.

12. Place diaphragm of the stethoscope over site where strongest beat is felt and apply moderate pressure with fingers of nondominant hand.

13. Begin to deflate cuff slowly by turning the thumbscrew counter-clockwise until the first beat is auscultated, usually about 3 mm Hg per second (this is the systolic reading).

14. Continue to deflate cuff slowly and note readings at Korotkoff sounds especially the fourth and fifth to determine diastolic reading.

15. When sounds are no longer heard, deflate cuff to 0 and remove.

16. If reading is questioned and blood pressure procedure is to be repeated, wait 30 seconds, raise arm before reinflating and return to level position with heart and repeat as outlined in the above procedure steps beginning with #11.

17. Continue with respirations, pulse and temperature, if appropriate, and make resident comfortable.

❧ PROBLEM-SOLVING ACTIONS

1. Monitor blood pressure while at rest; hurrying through procedure may alter pressure measurement.

2. Support arm that has clothing removed when applying cuff and avoid using arm that has an intravenous infusion in place or is on the same side that a mastectomy has been performed.

3. Monitor blood pressure at frequency dictated by disorder and medical regimen.

4. The amount of pressure exerted against the artery by the stethoscope diaphragm affects the measurement of the blood pressure, and if excessive, may obliterate the sound altogether.

5. The Korotkoff sounds are divided into 5 phases with differences in pitch and intensity with diastolic readings at fourth or fifth sounds.

6. If the auscultatory method is not possible, palpation of the pulsations may be used as the cuff is released to determine the systolic pressure. The diastolic may not be palpable.

7. Systolic readings in the use of the popliteal site are 10 to 40 mm Hg higher than those obtained at the brachial site with the diastolic readings about the same.

8. Note orders for monitoring blood pressure in both arms, sitting, standing, or lying positions.

9. The same extremity/position should be used for serial measurements to prevent variation in readings.

❧ EVALUATION

Blood pressure within baseline parameters, optimal effects of antihypertensive medications achieved

BLOOD PRESSURE, STANDING/SITTING

*T*he blood pressure taken in the standing and sitting position is measured to determine the heart's ability to adapt to position changes as revealed by changes in the pressure readings. The brachial site is used whenever possible to obtain measurements for comparison of the readings in these two positions.

❧ ASSESSMENT

Blood pressure range and pulse pressure, presence of dizziness when moving from a lying to sitting or standing position, presence of cardiovascular instability, hypertension or hypotension

❧ NURSING DIAGNOSES

High Risk for Trauma; Altered Tissue Perfusion (Cerebral)

❧ GOALS

Blood pressure measurement within established baseline parameters with position changes; correct monitoring of brachial blood pressure in standing/sitting position

❧ INTERVENTIONS

Equipment/Supplies

- Mercury or aneroid sphygmomanometer with cuff of appropriate size
- Antiseptic sponge
- Stethoscope

Resident

- Explain purpose of procedure and expected results
- Place in position of rest in lying position initially, change to sitting and standing position when appropriate with antecubital space exposed on one arm

❧ PROCEDURE

1. Perform handwashing.
2. Become familiar with baseline blood pressure readings to serve as a comparison in the three different positions (lying, standing, and sitting).
3. Perform blood pressure procedure in lying position (see procedure for Blood Pressure, Brachial) to note a baseline for comparison.
4. Assist the resident in assuming a sitting position at side of bed.
5. Allow to rest for 1 minute and take blood pressure again.
6. Assist the resident to a standing position and take blood pressure again.
7. Note changes in the three different positions.
8. Assist resident to bed or position of comfort.

❧ PROBLEM-SOLVING ACTIONS

1. Allow any dizziness or faintness to subside when assuming a sitting or standing position before taking blood pressure or changing positions.

2. Monitor blood pressure in these positions at frequency dictated by disorder and physician order.

3. Offer assistance for position changes to resident who is unstable or debilitated.

❧ EVALUATION

Variations in blood pressure within baseline parameters regardless of position changes

HEIGHT AND WEIGHT, STANDING/BED/CHAIR

Height and weight (Ht/Wt) measurements are included in the general assessment of a resident as an indicator of fluid and nutritional status. Tables of desired weights based on height, sex, age and frame are available to determine overweight or underweight, as well as gains and losses that occur during an illness or over a period of time during a chronic illness. Height and weight measurements are often important in calculating amounts of medications to be prescribed and administered. Height is usually taken once while weight may be monitored as frequently as once a day or week depending on reason for the procedure.

❧ ASSESSMENT

Medications taken that may affect weight gain or loss (diuretic or steroid), medical condition that affects food intake or utilization, (anorexia, vomiting, diarrhea), amounts of weight gain or weight loss

❧ NURSING DIAGNOSES

Altered Nutrition: Less Than Body Requirements; Altered Nutrition: More Than Body Requirements; High Risk for Fluid Volume Deficit or Excess

❧ GOALS

Maintenance of optimal weight based on standards according to age, sex, frame and height; correct monitoring of weight, fluid and nutritional status

❧ INTERVENTIONS

Equipment/Supplies

- Tape measure, yardstick, or height attachment on a standing scale
- Upright or bathroom scale for standing weight
- Chair scale for sitting weight

- Bed scale for weight in supine position

- Protector for scale (paper towel for standing or blanket/plastic cover for chair scales)

Resident

- Explain purpose of procedure and expected results
- Provide robe and slippers or appropriate drape depending on type of scale used

- Standing, sitting or supine position depending on client condition and abilities

❧ PROCEDURE

1. Perform handwashing.
2. Become familiar with charts listing normal weight for resident based on age, sex, frame and height or any established baselines in height and weight of resident.
3. Determine type of scale and/or measuring device needed based on resident's condition.
4. If resident is able to stand:
   a. Balance upright scale.
   b. Place paper towel on scale.

   c. Remove shoes and assist resident to stand erect on scale; cover scale with paper towel.

   d. Raise attachment to measure height above head of resident.

   e. Lower attachment to top of resident's head and note measurement as calibrated on the measuring device in inches or centimeters.

   f. Remove attachment device from top of resident's head and adjust or balance scale at zero for weight measurement on both arms of the scale.

   g. Note weight measurement at point of balance on arm of the scale calibrated in pounds or kilograms.

   h. Return scale to neutral state.

   i. Assist resident off scale, replace slippers, robe or other clothing, return to room.

5. If resident is able to sit but not stand:

   a. Cover chair with blanket or plastic protective cover, lock the scale and unlock arm if present.

   b. Balance chair scale.

   c. Remove shoes and assist resident to sit on chair scale with the arm open; close and lock in place after resident comfortably seated.

   d. Adjust scale for weight measurement on both arms of the scale.

   e. Note weight measurement at point of balance on arm of the scale calibrated in pounds or kilograms.

   f. Return scale to neutral state, unlock arm and open.

   g. Assist resident off scale, replace slippers and clothing, return to room via wheelchair.

6. If resident is not able to sit or stand:

   a. Place in supine position with knees straight and arms straight at sides of body.

   b. Using a tape measuring device, measure from the top of the head to the sole of the foot at right angle to the leg; mark the sheet at the top and bottom as tape measure is not long enough.

   c. Note measurement as calibrated on the device in inches or centimeters.

   d. Place bed scale next to the side of the bed, place resident in sidelying position with back towards scale.

   e. Lower board and lock, lock brakes on scale and pump handle to raise board above mattress level.

   f. Balance bed scale weight gauge at zero and center beam.

   g. Lower board using the release flat on the bed and place resident on the board (obtain assistance if needed).

   h. Pump handle to raise boards slightly above mattress level; note that resident's body does not touch bed.

   i. Note weight measurement by reading beam or digital number depending on type of bed scale used, calibration in pounds or kilograms.

   j. Release lift to place board on bed and place resident back on bed.

   k. Raise board high enough to clear mattress, release brake and remove scale from bedside.

   l. Unlock board and return to upright position and lock in place.

   m. Position resident for comfort and replace linens for warmth.

   n. Remove scale from room to place of storage.

❧ PROBLEM-SOLVING ACTIONS

1. Height may be noted in centimeters or feet and inches or converted using the equivalency of 1 inch = 2.54 cm.

2. Weight may be noted in kilograms or pounds and ounces or converted using the equivalency of 1 kilogram = 2.2 pounds, or 1 kilogram = 1000 grams, or 1 pound = 453. 6 grams, or 1 ounce = 30 grams.

3. Height should be measured to the nearest ¼ inch.

4. Weight should be measured to the nearest ¼ pound or 0.1 kilogram; ½ ounce or 10 grams.

5. Weigh resident on same scale, at same time of day (preferably morning) while wearing the same amount of clothing.

6. A lifting sheet may be used to place resident on bed scale board but the weight of the sheet should be deducted from the resident's weight reading.

7. Skin fold measurements may be performed for additional data regarding weight changes and amount of body fat in obese residents.

&. EVALUATION

Weight maintained within baseline parameters, weight gains or losses of less than 10 to 20 percent for ideal height and frame, age and sex, medical disorder and general condition

PULSE, APICAL

The apical pulse is the heartbeat heard at the apex of the heart with the use of a stethoscope. The apex is the site used to obtain a pulse when the radial pulse reveals abnormal characteristics and when medications affecting heart function are administered. The apical pulse is also included in the assessment of heart sounds during physical examination of the cardiovascular system. Performing this procedure simultaneously with a radial pulse may determine the pulse deficit. The radial pulse is usually 1-2 beats less than the apical, and this deficit often signals a problem with circulatory status. An apical pulse is counted for one full minute with rate, rhythm and quality of the heartbeat noted.

❧ ASSESSMENT

Rate, rhythm, and quality of heartbeat, presence of irregularities or arrhythmias, administration of cardiac glycosides to determine need to withhold medication

❧ NURSING DIAGNOSES

Decreased Cardiac Output; Altered Tissue Perfusion (Cardiopulmonary, Cerebral, Renal, Gastrointestinal, Peripheral)

❧ GOALS

Apical pulse rate, rhythm, quality within established baseline parameters; correct monitoring of apical pulse and cardiovascular status

❧ INTERVENTIONS

Equipment/Supplies

- Watch with a second hand
- Stethoscope
- Antiseptic sponge

Resident

- Explain purpose of procedure and expected results
- Place in supine position with left chest exposed and other body parts draped for privacy and warmth

❧ PROCEDURE

1. Perform handwashing.
2. Become familiar with baseline apical pulse characteristics and cardiovascular status that serve as an indication for monitoring.
3. Become aware of cardiac medications ordered and assessment required prior to administration.
4. Cleanse ear tips of stethoscope and place in ears, diaphragm of the stethoscope can also be cleansed.
5. Identify the midclavicular line with the fingers of the nondominant hand (warm hands by rubbing together).
6. Using the same hand, palpate the intercostal spaces with the finger pads to the fifth space and move hand and fingers over this area to locate apical beat.
7. Warm diaphragm and place over the apical area with the dominant hand and hold in place.

8. Auscultate for the sound (lub-dub) of the heartbeat.

9. Count beats for 60 seconds with each lub-dub signifying a single beat and note rhythm and quality and any deviations from baseline values.

10. After completing count, remove drape, replace gown or clothing and leave resident in a comfortable state.

❧ PROBLEM-SOLVING ACTIONS

1. Monitor apical pulse while at rest as anxiety, activity, or external stimuli will affect rate.

2. Monitor pulse at frequency dictated by condition or medication regimen.

3. Counting heartbeat for exactly 60 seconds.

4. Change position to left sidelying if unable to hear beat in supine position.

5. Concentrate on the sound of the beat and avoid listening to other chest sounds that may interfere.

❧ EVALUATION

Apical pulse within baseline parameters, optimal rate maintained with medications given for cardiac condition

PULSE, APICAL/RADIAL

*T*he apical/radial pulse is obtained by counting the beats at these two sites simultaneously for a full minute by two people; one palpating the radial pulse and one auscultating the apical pulse. The difference between the two counts, if any, is the pulse deficit. The deficit indicates that a heartbeat (contraction) does not have the strength to cause a palpable pulse at a peripheral site. If two people are not available, an accurate rate cannot be determined for both pulses, but one person may palpate the radial pulse while auscultating the apical pulse to evaluate if the rates are approximately the same or if any discrepancies exist.

ASSESSMENT

Rate, rhythm, and quality of apical/radial pulses and presence of deficit, presence of atrial fibrillation or premature ventricular contractions which may result in deficit

NURSING DIAGNOSES

Altered Cardiac Output; Altered Tissue Perfusion (Cardiopulmonary, Peripheral)

GOALS

Apical/radial pulse rate, rhythm, quality within established baseline parameters; apical/radial pulse rate the same; correct monitoring of apical/radial pulse

INTERVENTIONS

Equipment/Supplies

- Watch with a second hand
- Stethoscope
- Antiseptic sponge
- Second person

Resident

- Explain purpose of procedure and expected results
- Place in supine position with right chest, hand and wrist exposed and other body parts draped for privacy and warmth

PROCEDURE

1. Perform handwashing.
2. Become familiar with baseline apical/radial pulse characteristics and deficit, cardiovascular status.
3. Decide who will take the apical and who will take the radial pulse.
4. Place watch with second hand within view of both persons performing the procedure.
5. Each person locates respective sites (see Pulse, Apical and Pulse, Radial).
6. When both persons are ready, one signals the time to start count and end count after exactly 60 seconds.
7. Note rate, rhythm and quality and any deviations from baseline values.
8. Compare the two counts and determine if a deficit is present.
9. After completion of counts, remove drape, replace gown or clothing and leave resident in a comfortable position.

❧ PROBLEM-SOLVING ACTIONS

1. Monitor apical/radial pulse while at rest as activity or external stimuli will affect rates.
2. Monitor pulses at frequency dictated by condition or deficit.
3. Start counting simultaneously when time begins and end count exactly at 60 seconds. Determine who will signal the times in advance.
4. Repeat counts if deficit is more than 2 beats or if accuracy of the procedure is in question.

❧ EVALUATION

Apical/radial pulse within baseline parameters, deficit limited to 1 or 2 beats

PULSE, PERIPHERAL

Peripheral pulses indicate whether or not there is adequate circulation to the extremities. They are monitored to assess the vascular competency and tissue perfusion of the arms, legs, and feet, especially when the resident's age and medical condition cause changes in the blood vessels. Sites are the femoral artery in the groin area, popliteal artery behind the knee, brachial artery in the antecubital space, and dorsalis pedis artery in the dorsal aspect of the foot. Specific needs determine which peripheral site is used to obtain the pulse.

ASSESSMENT

Pulse rate/minute with rhythm, quality of beat, presence of circulatory disorder affecting extremities or risk for circulatory problem; presence of any restrictive devices, such as restraints, casts, or traction

NURSING DIAGNOSES

Activity Intolerance; Altered Tissue Perfusion (Peripheral)

GOALS

Peripheral pulse rate, rhythm, quality and pattern within established baseline parameters; correct monitoring of appropriate pulse and circulatory status of extremity

INTERVENTIONS

Equipment/Supplies

- Watch with a second hand
- Doppler stethoscope if needed

Resident

- Explain purpose of procedure and expected results
- Place in position to expose area of pulse to be used and drape accordingly for privacy and warmth

PROCEDURE

1. Perform handwashing.
2. Become familiar with baseline peripheral pulse and characteristics and circulatory status of the extremities to serve as a comparison.
3. Palpate for pulse at site to be used with pads of middle and forefinger as follows:
   a. For femoral, in supine position with palpation of groin area on both sides and compare, noting rate, rhythm, and quality during compression against ischium.
   b. For popliteal, in supine or prone position with knee flexed and palpation of back of knee slightly lateral noting rate, rhythm and quality during compression against femur.
   c. For brachial, in supine position and palpation of the antecubital space, noting rate, rhythm and quality during compression against ulna.
   d. For dorsalis pedis, in supine or sitting position with foot at 90 degree angle to lower leg and palpation of dorsal aspect between first and second toe noting rate, rhythm, and quality during compression against phalanges.
4. Using the second hand on the watch, count the number of beats occurring in 30 seconds and calculate the rate for one full minute (multiply by 2).

5. Count for a full minute if abnormal characteristics are noted or repeat if necessary to obtain the correct information.

6. Note any deviation from baseline values in rate, rhythm, quality and pattern.

7. After completing count, remove drape, replace gown or clothing and leave resident in comfortable state.

❧ PROBLEM-SOLVING ACTIONS

1. Monitor pulse while at rest and with area properly positioned.

2. Monitor pulse at frequency dictated by disorder and condition of resident.

3. Support area when taking pulse as muscular contractions caused by trying to support limb affect pulse.

4. Start counting pulse when time begins and count for exactly 60 seconds.

5. The dorsalis pedis pulse may be congenitally absent and, therefore, not be available as a site for monitoring.

6. The amount of pressure exerted against the artery affects the quality and rhythm of the pulse and, if excessive, may obliterate the pulse altogether.

7. Take pulses on both sides or extremities and compare for differences in evaluating peripheral pulses.

8. If pulse is difficult to obtain, consider use of a Doppler stethoscope, if available.

9. Consider temperature and color of skin of extremity as signs of impaired circulation, tissue perfusion associated with pulse changes.

❧ EVALUATION

Peripheral pulse taken within baseline parameters, optimal rate maintained and circulatory status of extremities maintained

PULSE, RADIAL

Pulse (P) is the beat or wave felt at a superficial arterial site that results from the heart forcing the blood from the left ventricle into the circulation. The radial pulse is monitored routinely to determine baselines and changes in rate, rhythm, quality, and pattern. The number of beats occurring in one minute constitute the pulse rate. The rhythm is the presence of regular or irregular beats. Pulse quality and pattern reflects the strength of the pulse indicating the volume of blood pumped by the heart contraction. The radial pulse is usually taken at the same time as respirations, blood pressure and temperature measurements. Other superficial sites for monitoring arterial pulse include temporal, carotid, brachial, femoral, popliteal, and dorsalis pedis. These sites may be used when the radial site is not available for use or to monitor peripheral pulses in the arms, legs and feet.

ASSESSMENT

Pulse rate/minute with presence of tachycardia or bradycardia, rhythm and pattern as bigeminy, regular or irregular, and fibrillation; quality (amplitude) as strong, weak or bounding, presence of cardiovascular disease causing alteration in pulse

NURSING DIAGNOSES

Decreased Cardiac Output; Activity Intolerance; Altered Tissue Perfusion (Cardiopulmonary, Cerebral, Renal, Gastrointestinal); Fluid Volume Deficit

GOALS

Pulse rate, rhythm, quality and pattern within established baseline parameters; correct monitoring of radial pulse and cardiovascular status

INTERVENTIONS

Equipment/Supplies

- Watch with a second hand

Resident

- Explain purpose of procedure and expected results

- Place in position of rest and comfort, lying or sitting with hand and wrist exposed and relaxed with palm in pronation

PROCEDURE

1. Perform handwashing.
2. Become familiar with baseline pulse characteristics and cardiovascular status to serve as a comparison.
3. Palpate for radial pulse at wrist site on thumb side with pads of middle and forefinger, avoid using thumb because the pulse at this site may be mistaken for the resident's pulse.
4. After locating the pulse beat, apply moderate pressure to the area where the strongest beat is felt as the artery is compressed against the radius.
5. Using the second hand on the watch, count the number of beats occurring in 15 or 30 seconds if the rate is regular and calculate the rate for one minute (multiply by 4 if 15 seconds or 2 if 30 seconds).

6. Count the pulse for one full minute if abnormal characteristics are noted, repeat if necessary to obtain the correct rate.

7. Note any deviations from baseline values in rate, rhythm, quality and pattern.

8. Next count respirations, then leave resident in comfortable position.

❧ PROBLEM-SOLVING ACTIONS

1. Monitor pulse while at rest as anxiety, activity or external stimuli will affect rate.

2. Monitor pulse at a frequency dictated by disorder and condition of the resident.

3. Provide support to arm when taking pulse because muscular contractions may alter pulse rate.

4. Start counting pulse when time begins and end count at exactly 60 seconds.

5. The amount of pressure exerted against the artery affects the quality and rhythm of the pulse and, if excessive, may obliterate the pulse altogether.

6. If unable to obtain an accurate pulse, take an apical pulse using a stethoscope.

❧ EVALUATION

Pulse within baseline parameters; optimal circulatory status maintained

RESPIRATIONS

Respiration (R) is the process of inspiration (taking in oxygen) and expiration (removal of carbon dioxide and other wastes) needed to sustain body functions. The monitoring of respirations is done routinely to determine baselines and detect changes in the respiratory rate, rhythm, depth, ease and pattern. A respiration is 1 inspiration and 1 expiration, and the number of respirations occurring in one minute constitutes the respiratory rate. The rhythm and ease of respirations are the interval equality between each inspiration/expiration cycle and the effort expended during this process. Respiratory depth is the amount of air inspired and expired in each cycle and the pattern includes characteristics such as difficulty in breathing, slowness, rapidity of breathing, or periodic absence of breathing. Respirations are usually taken with pulse, blood pressure and temperature measurements.

⋙ ASSESSMENT

Respiratory rate/minute with presence of tachypnea or bradycardia, rhythm as regular or irregular, depth as shallow or deep or presence of hyperpnea, pattern as apnea, dyspnea, orthopnea, hyperventilation, hypoventilation, sound as wheezing, stridor, presence of cyanosis, use of accessory muscles, respiratory disease causing alterations in respirations

⋙ NURSING DIAGNOSES

Ineffective Breathing Pattern; Ineffective Airway Clearance, Impaired Gas Exchange; Activity Intolerance; Fluid Volume Excess

⋙ GOALS

Respiratory rate, rhythm, depth, ease, and pattern within established baseline parameters; correct monitoring of respiratory status

⋙ INTERVENTIONS

Equipment/Supplies

- Watch with a second hand
- Stethoscope

Resident

- Explain purpose of procedure and expected results
- Place in position of comfort, either supine with chest in full view, or in cases of respiratory difficulty, semi or high Fowler's

⋙ PROCEDURE

1. Perform handwashing.
2. Become familiar with baseline respiratory status to serve as a comparison.
3. After taking the pulse, leave fingers on wrist while observing chest movement and monitoring respirations.
4. Count the rise and fall of the chest for 30 seconds, if regular, and multiply by 2 or for 1 full minute if irregular in rhythm.
5. Note other characteristics or deviations from baseline values in pattern or sounds.

6. Auscultate breath sounds with stethoscope if abnormal breath sounds are audible or other abnormal characteristics of breathing are present.

7. Reposition and leave in comfortable, restful position.

PROBLEM-SOLVING ACTIONS

1. Monitor respirations while resident is at rest as anxiety or activity will affect breathing pattern.

2. Remove clothing from waist up if difficult to observe chest movement.

3. In those who experience respiratory difficulty, position for optimal breathing and chest expansion before taking respirations.

4. Palpate chest for symmetry and movement during respiration if visualization is difficult.

5. Monitor respirations at frequency dictated by disorder and condition of resident.

EVALUATION

Respirations within baseline parameters, adequate gas exchange and airway patency

TEMPERATURE, ORAL/AXILLARY/RECTAL/AURAL WITH ELECTRONIC THERMOMETER

Temperature (T) is the body heat produced by body processes with consideration of heat losses into the environment from the skin, lungs, and waste materials. Monitoring of the temperature is done routinely to determine baselines and changes, including increases and decreases associated with health status. Determinations can be made in Celsius (C) or Fahrenheit (F) scales of measurement and taken by the oral, axillary, aural or rectal routes. The oral and aural routes are the most common. The axillary, and rectal routes are used when the oral or aural routes are contraindicated because of injury or trauma, or in an uncooperative or cognitively-impaired resident. The axillary route is the least accurate and should only be used when the temperature cannot be obtained by other routes. Methods of obtaining a temperature include the use of a mercury glass thermometer, electronic thermometer, a disposable thermometer, or disposable chemical dot thermometer. Normal values for temperatures vary with route used for measurement. The electronic method takes a temperature reading in a shorter period of time than the mercury thermometer procedure (usually by 30 seconds). It utilizes a probe with a sensing tip and a readout of numbers on the thermometer unit panel.

❧ ASSESSMENT

Temperature readings with increase or decrease, route and time of day, factors present that affect body temperature, presence of disorder that predisposes to temperature changes

❧ NURSING DIAGNOSES

Hyperthermia; Hypothermia

❧ GOALS

Temperature within established baseline parameters for route used; correct monitoring of temperature and health status

❧ INTERVENTIONS

Equipment/Supplies

- Electronic thermometer with probe connected to thermometer unit and a base for charging
- Container of disposable probes
- Aural electronic temperature device with disposable tips

- Lubricant for rectal probe

- Tissues

Resident

- Explain purpose of procedure and expected results

- Place in position of comfort, lying in supine position or sitting for oral, aural and axillary route with axilla exposed, lying in side-lying position with buttocks exposed and draped appropriately for rectal route

❧ PROCEDURE

1. Perform handwashing.

2. Become familiar with baseline temperature, route used and time of day measured to serve as a comparison.

3. Remove the thermometer unit from the base and carry to resident.

4. Hold probe with dominant hand and insert into a disposable cover in the box; use proper probes and covers for oral and rectal measurements, axillary uses the same as oral.

5. Follow the steps for measurement of temperature by oral, axillary, or rectal with mercury thermometer except that the probe is only inserted ¼-½ inches for rectal route.

6. Insert the tip of the aural electronic device into the external canal of the ear.

7. When probe is in place, note readout of temperature in digits on the panel until a light appears indicating that temperature has been reached.

8. Note readout that is registered in whole numbers and tenths of numbers.

9. Remove probe from the site used and push the button on the probe to eject the cover and discard.

10. Replace the thermometer into the charging base and return the probe to its holder.

11. Return resident to position of comfort.

❧ PROBLEM-SOLVING ACTIONS

1. Normally, higher temperatures are noted in the late afternoon and evening and lower temperatures in the early morning.

2. The same route and same times of day should be used to monitor temperature as normal values vary with routes.

3. Dentures should be removed for oral measurement.

4. A period of 15 minutes should be allowed to elapse before taking temperature if hot or cold fluid has been ingested, a hot bath or shower taken, smoking or excessive activity has been performed, room temperature fluctuates, or mouth breathing or gum chewing has been noted.

5. Monitor temperature at frequency dictated by a disorder or condition of the resident (flushed, chilled, shivering, warm or hot or cold skin).

6. Retake temperature if accuracy is questioned; wait 5 minutes before repeating procedure.

❧ EVALUATION

Temperature maintained within baseline parameters for route used and time of day monitored, environmental factors that affect temperature controlled or eliminated

TEMPERATURE, ORAL/AXILLARY/RECTAL WITH MERCURY THERMOMETER

Temperature (T) is the body heat produced by the body processes with the consideration of heat losses into the environment from the skin, lungs and waste products. The monitoring of the temperature is done routinely to determine baselines and changes including increases and decreases associated with health status. Determinations may be made in Celsius or Fahrenheit scales of measurement (C and F, respectively) and taken by the oral, axillary, or rectal routes with the oral route being the most common. The heat pocket in the mouth serves as a constant source of arterial circulation for temperature measurement. The axillary or rectal sites are used when the oral route is contraindicated because of injury, risk of trauma from the thermometer in uncooperative or cognitively impaired residents. Methods of obtaining a temperature include a mercury thermometer, electronic thermometer, or disposable chemical dot thermometer. Normal values for temperatures vary with route used for measurement.

ASSESSMENT

Temperature readings with increase or decrease, route and time of day, factors present that affect body temperature, presence of disorder that predisposes to temperature changes

NURSING DIAGNOSES

Hyperthermia, Hypothermia

GOALS

Temperature within established baseline parameters for route used; correct monitoring of temperature and health status

INTERVENTIONS

Equipment/Supplies

- Mercury glass thermometer
- Water soluble lubricant
- Tissue wipes

- Mild soap and warm water for cleansing glass thermometer
- Antiseptic sponge
- Disposable gloves

Resident

- Explain purpose of procedure and expected results

- Place in position of comfort, lying in supine position or sitting for oral and axillary route with axilla exposed, lying in sidelying position with buttocks exposed and draped appropriately for rectal route

PROCEDURE

1. Perform handwashing.
2. Become familiar with baseline temperature, route used, and time of day measured to serve as a comparison.

3. For thermometer stored in a solution, remove and while holding the end without the mercury tip, wipe with tissue from fingers towards the mercury end; thermometer that is stored dry will not need to be wiped.

4. Continue holding the thermometer firmly in the dominant hand and briskly shake down using a wrist action to a reading of 96°F (35°C) or below.

5. Inspect thermometer for cracks or defects and obtain a new thermometer if needed.

6. If oral route is used:
   a. Ask resident to open mouth and raise the tongue.
   b. Insert the mercury end of the thermometer into the heat pocket under and towards the back of the tongue.
   c. Ask resident to close lips but not to bite the thermometer.
   d. Leave in place for 8 to 11 minutes.
   e. Remain in attendance if appropriate.
   f. Remove thermometer from mouth and hold at eye level to read calibration.
   g. Rotate the thermometer if necessary to obtain the reading.
   h. Note measurement and if changes are evident.
   i. Wash thermometer with soap and water, dry with tissue, wipe or replace in antiseptic solution.

7. If axillary route is used:
   a. Dry axillary area with a towel or tissue.
   b. Insert the mercury end of the thermometer into the axillary area and lower arm with the thermometer in place.
   c. Hold end of thermometer if needed to anchor in place.
   d. Leave in place for 10 minutes.
   e. Remain in attendance if appropriate.
   f. Remove thermometer from axilla by holding end and raising resident's arm.
   g. Hold thermometer at eye level to read calibration, rotate the thermometer if necessary to obtain the reading.
   h. Note measurement and if changes are evident.
   i. Wash thermometer with soap and water, dry with tissue wipe or replace in antiseptic solution.

8. If rectal route is used:
   a. Lubricate 1 to 2 inches of the mercury end of thermometer; put on gloves.
   b. Separate buttocks with nondominant hand and expose rectal area.
   c. Touch rectal area with bulb of thermometer and gently insert 1½-2 inches into the rectum in an upward direction; ask resident to take a deep breath through mouth to relax sphincter.
   d. Hold in place after releasing the buttocks for 3 to 4 minutes.
   e. Remove the thermometer and wipe with tissue from fingers to mercury bulb area with enough friction to allow visualization of the calibrations.
   f. Hold thermometer at eye level to read, rotate if necessary to obtain reading.
   g. Note measurement and if changes are evident.
   h. Wipe rectal area with tissue and return resident to position of comfort.
   i. Wash thermometer with soap and water, dry with tissue wipe or place in antiseptic solution.

✢ PROBLEM-SOLVING ACTIONS

1. Temperature is calibrated in two-tenths on the mercury thermometer.

2. Normally, higher temperatures are noted in the late afternoon and evening and lower temperatures in the early morning.

3. Dentures should be removed for oral temperatures.

4. Environmental factors which affect temperature include monitoring after a hot bath or shower, smoking, excessive activity, room/air temperature, ingestion of hot fluids, chewing gum, ingestion of cold fluids, and during oxygen administration; wait at least 15 minutes before taking temperature if these conditions exist.

5. Disposable sheaths may be used with mercury glass thermometers.

6. Rectal temperatures may be affected by stool in the rectum, presence of hemorrhoids that cause pain and trauma, or the possibility that the stimulation of the insertion of the thermometer may cause vagal stimulation resulting in bradycardia.

7. Perform axillary measurement when resident is disoriented or uncooperative, has injury or stomatitis of the oral cavity, or following surgery in oral cavity.

8. Monitor temperature at frequency dictated by disorder or condition of the resident (flushed, chilled, shivering, warm or hot or cold skin).

9. Methods of disinfection of thermometers as well as storage varies in agencies although the CDC recommends that each resident has own thermometer that is washed before and after each use and disinfected with 70% alcohol.

10. If the accuracy of the temperature is in question, retake the temperature using another thermometer.

11. Use right thermometer for right route as imprinted on the thermometer as Oral or Rectal.

❧ EVALUATION

Temperature maintained within baseline parameters for route used and time of day monitored, environmental factors that affect temperature controlled or eliminated

UNIT IV

PERSONAL HYGIENE

- Backrub
- Bath, Cooling Sponge
- Bath, Sitz
- Bath, Tub/Shower
- Bed, Occupied
- Bed, Unoccupied
- Bedbath, Complete
- Dentures
- Dressing/Personal Grooming
- Eye Glasses/Contact Lenses
- Eye Management of the Unconscious Resident

- Eye Prosthesis
- Foot Management
- Hair, Grooming/Shampoo
- Hearing Aids
- Nail Management
- Oral /Teeth Management
- Oral Management of the Unconscious Resident
- Perineal Management
- Shaving, Electric/Safety Razors
- Vaginal Irrigation

BACKRUB

The backrub massage promotes relaxation, skin integrity, stimulation of circulation and muscular activity, and allows for therapeutic touch. The use of massage soothes the skin and makes it more pliable and tougher, stimulates muscles, prevents atrophy, and stimulates the circulation to improve nutrition and elimination of wastes. The areas massaged can include the neck, back, buttocks, and shoulders. Various movements are employed during a backrub, such as, stroking, effleurage, kneading, friction, and tapotement, each applied at a consistent rhythm and rate. It can be done following a bath for comfort, during periods of stress to reduce anxiety, or at bedtime to promote sleep. The procedure is especially helpful to residents who are bedridden or physically limited for activities or movement.

ASSESSMENT

Skin condition at bony prominences and possible decubitus ulcer formation, allergies to massage lotions or lubricants, possible contraindication to massage, muscular fatigue, obesity or emaciation, bedrest and activity status

NURSING DIAGNOSES

Anxiety; High Risk for Activity Intolerance; High Risk for Impaired Skin Integrity; Sleep Pattern Disturbance

GOALS

Improved skin integrity, endurance, and sleep; correct massage movements based on rationale for the procedure

INTERVENTIONS

Equipment/Supplies

- Basin of warm water, mild soap, washcloth and soft towel
- Bath blanket

- Skin lotion, lubricant, powder as needed
- Clean gown or pajamas

Resident

- Explain purpose of procedure and expected results
- Place in sidelying or prone position and drape to expose back and areas for massage

PROCEDURE

1. Perform handwashing.
2. Become familiar with the reason for the backrub and types of massage movements to be performed.
3. Wash and pat dry the back.
4. Warm the lotion or oil to promote relaxation and prevent vasoconstriction and muscle tension.
5. Place some lotion or oil on the hands and rub together.
6. Position yourself at the side of the bed in a stance that permits base of support and balance.
7. Massage the back and other areas using the following movements:
   a. Stroke using the entire palmar surfaces of the hands with fingers together and applying an equal

amount of pressure in long sweeping upward and outward movements depending on the reason for massage, such as, effleurage which is a light touch stroke that soothes and reduces muscle tension, deep stroking, which is an increase in the pressure to increase circulation.

b. Compress using more forceful movements, such as, kneading or petrissage done by grasping or compressing the muscle or skin fold by the thumb and fingers and then performing a circular motion as the pressure is tightened, loosened and finally released to enhance circulation; friction is done by applying pressure that is graduated from light to firm as the superficial tissue is moved over the deeper tissues with a circular movement by the palmar sides of the hand and fingers to stimulate circulation.

c. Tapotement using the ulnar border of the hands and percussion with short, gentle blows or tapping on an area with the fingers or clapping an area with the fingers, or clapping an area with the fingers while the hand forms a cup-like shape to loosen secretions in the chest or stimulate muscle contraction.

8. Remove excess lotion or oil from the area at the conclusion of the massage with towel.

9. Change the gown and any soiled linens if needed.

10. Place resident in position of comfort; remove, clean, and store articles for future use.

❧ PROBLEM-SOLVING ACTIONS

1. Massage movements at the rate of 15/minute and a limit of 10 minutes for back massage is recommended to prevent a hyperemic reaction of the skin and muscles.

2. Effleurage stroking can be done at the start and end of the massage procedure to relieve muscle tension.

3. Massage of the extremities is contraindicated in those on bedrest because of the vulnerability to thrombus formation or to any area that has had trauma to superficial or deep tissue because of the possibility of increased damage or hemorrhage.

4. Talcum powder should not be used on the dry skin common to the elderly; oils (mineral, coconut, glycerin) and lotions should be selected for their lubricating effect.

5. Assessment of skin and muscle status, especially in those who are obese, emaciated or are on bedrest should be done during the backrub.

6. Place the resident as close to the edge of the bed as possible to perform backrub.

7. Avoid pressure massage of bony areas with very little muscle tissue covering.

❧ EVALUATION

Rest and sleep promoted; skin intact and free from reddened areas; anxiety/stress reduced and relaxation improved

BATH, COOLING SPONGE

The cooling sponge bath is a wet cold application performed to reduce body temperature when the individual has a fever. It involves the use of tepid water, or a mixture of water and alcohol at 80-93° F. It dilates superficial blood vessels and releases heat from the skin surfaces by evaporation. Lower temperatures of the water will cause vasoconstriction of the vessels which reduces the peripheral circulation and inhibits the transfer of heat to the skin. It may not be an effective treatment in the elderly with vascular diseases that impair circulation or for those who have unstable vital signs. For this reason, and the availability of antipyretic and antibiotic therapy to treat elevated temperatures, this procedure has limited use in residents over 60 years of age.

ASSESSMENT

Elevated temperature, chills, diaphoresis, age, signs and symptoms of infectious process

NURSING DIAGNOSES

High Risk for Altered Body Temperature; Hyperthermia

GOAL

Body temperature maintained within normal baseline ranges

INTERVENTIONS

Equipment/Supplies

- Basin of tepid water
- Half-strength alcohol in water
- Bath thermometer
- Towels and washcloth
- Hot water bottle and cover
- Thermometer, mercury/electronic
- Bath blankets
- Bed protector

Resident

- Explain purpose of procedure and expected results
- Warm, draft free environment
- Place in supine position

PROCEDURE

1. Perform handwashing.
2. Become familiar with pattern of temperature elevation, reason to perform cooling sponge bath, possible response to procedure (chilling, shivering).
3. Place bed protectors under the resident and cover with bath blankets.
4. Take rectal temperature and pulse to establish a baseline.
5. Sponge the face with moist washcloth and pat dry. Expose and sponge each body part except chest and abdomen for 5 minutes and cover with the bath blanket without drying.
6. Place a wet washcloth on the forehead, at both axillae, and at the groin to enhance heat loss.

7. Place a warm water bottle at the feet to help prevent shivering.

8. Monitor pulse periodically during the procedure to note tolerance.

9. Continue the procedure for 30 minutes by rotating the areas and including the back and buttocks if tolerated.

10. Change water and washcloths to maintain desirable temperature.

11. Continue to measure temperature and pulse following the procedure for 45 minutes; repeat procedure if temperature remains elevated.

12. Pat dry body parts and position for comfort and care.

13. Remove, cleanse, and discard or store equipment and supplies used.

❧ PROBLEM-SOLVING ACTIONS

1. Avoid areas near the genitalia when using alcohol in the water.

2. All parts of the body should be covered except the area being sponged.

3. Note changes such as mottling, nail or lip cyanosis, chills, shivering, changes in pulse, and stop the procedure immediately.

4. A moist towel can be substituted for a washcloth to sponge larger areas.

5. Administration of an antipyretic prior to the procedure can be beneficial in reducing temperature.

6. Rectal temperature monitoring is preferred for more accurate readings if this is permitted for an individual resident.

7. Frequency of linen changes should depend on resident's comfort, endurance, and activity tolerance; protective pads can be used to control frequency if incontinence is a problem.

8. Gloves should be worn if the linens are soiled with blood or body fluids.

9. When linens are removed, they should be observed for dentures or other prostheses to prevent loss of these articles.

❧ EVALUATION

Reduction in temperature following cooling sponge bath

BATH, SITZ

The sitz bath is the immersion of the hips, buttocks and perineal in hot (98-104°F) or warm (96-98°F) water to achieve the beneficial effects of moist heat. It is done to provide continuous or intermittent treatments for pain, inflammation, or infection at the perineal area resulting from surgery or skin irritation caused by incontinence of urine and/or feces. The vasodilation that occurs from the effects of the heat promotes circulation to the area that facilitates comfort and healing. It can be performed with the use of the traditional bathtub, a permanent sitz bathtub, or a disposable plastic sitz bath with a drainage system that can be placed on the toilet seat. This system is connected to a container filled with water and tubing connected to the bath container, to provide a continuous and consistent temperature of water and drainage system into the toilet.

ASSESSMENT

Condition of the perineal area skin, secretions, itching or pain, irritation, disruption in skin integrity, presence of a urinary catheter or dressings

NURSING DIAGNOSES

High Risk for Infection; High Risk for Impaired Skin Integrity; Pain

GOAL

Promote pain relief and comfort by providing moist heat safely and appropriately

INTERVENTIONS

Equipment/Supplies

- Bathtub, permanent or portable sitz bath
- 2 bath towels, bath mat
- Stool or chair to sit on
- Bath thermometer
- Bath blanket
- IV pole as needed
- Plastic ring as appropriate

Resident

- Explain purpose of procedure and expected results
- Remove clothing, pajama bottom or gown from the waist down

PROCEDURE

1. Perform handwashing.
2. Offer the bedpan or urinal, or assist to void in bathroom prior to the procedure.
3. Become familiar with the type of bath equipment, temperature of water based on the purpose of the treatment.
4. Fill the tub or permanent sitz tub with water about a quarter full to cover buttocks, perineal area and adjust the temperature to 98-104°F depending on the purpose of the treatment and tolerance to the temperature.

5. If a disposable unit is used, lift the toilet seat and place in position, fill the bag hung on the IV pole above the height of the resident's head with water and adjust the temperature to 98-104°F, regulate the flow into the sitz bath with the clamp.

6. Place a folded towel, bath mat, or inflated ring if used in the bathtub for the resident to sit on to alleviate pressure to a painful area.

7. Assist into the tub or on the sitz tub; support knees and lumbar portion of the back with a folded towel and the feet with a stool if the disposable sitz tub is used.

8. Cover the resident with the bath blanket for privacy and warmth.

9. Take the pulse to serve as a baseline and every 5 minutes during the bath.

10. Allow the resident to remain in the sitz bath for 20 minutes unless weakness or pulse change is noted; remain if disabled or weak.

11. Check water temperature with the thermometer and add warm water when necessary to tub or bag hanging on the IV pole to maintain constant temperature.

12. Assess pulse, weakness, and dizziness at the end of the procedure and assist out of the bath or off the sitz bath container and pat the skin dry.

13. Assist to dress with clean gown or pajamas.

14. Dispose of used articles or place in the laundry hamper; empty, cleanse, and disinfect the tub or disposable sitz bath equipment for future use.

✷ PROBLEM-SOLVING ACTIONS

1. Avoid sitz bath treatment if resident is weak, debilitated, or has cardiovascular instability.

2. Monitor tolerance to the treatment to prevent untoward effects of vasodilation.

3. Place a call light within reach for resident to call for assistance if feeling weak or faint.

4. The permanent sitz bath or disposable sitz bath is preferred over the tub since vasodilation of the extremities removes circulation from the area being treated and reduces therapeutic value of the procedure.

5. Test the tolerance to the water temperature by allowing the resident to slowly sit down or place some of the water on the inner aspect of the thigh; assist to stand up or add cool water if water feels too hot; wait while water cools and assist to sit down again.

✷ EVALUATION

Improved comfort, circulation and healing of the perineal area

BATH, TUB/SHOWER

Bathing by tub bath or shower is done to remove soil, dead epithelial cells, microorganisms from the skin, and body odor to promote comfort, cleanliness, circulation, and relaxation. A medicated tub bath can also be provided to treat skin conditions. The aging skin becomes dry, wrinkled, thinner, and blemished with various aging spots over time and is easily affected by environmental temperature and humidity, sun exposure, soaps, and clothing fabrics. The frequency and type of bathing depends on resident preference, skin condition, tolerance and energy level. Although a daily bath or shower is preferred and necessary for some, the aging skin can be maintained by bathing every two days or with partial bathing as needed.

❧ ASSESSMENT

Usual pattern of bathing and ability to bathe independently, skin condition for color or pigmentation, texture, eruptions, irritations, pruritus, bruising, temperature, allergies to bathing products, presence of body odor, antihypertensive therapy

❧ NURSING DIAGNOSES

High Risk for Impaired Skin Integrity; Self-Care Deficit, Bathing; High Risk for Trauma

❧ GOALS

Maintenance of skin integrity, optimal level of comfort and cleanliness

❧ INTERVENTIONS

Equipment/Supplies

- Nonskid strips on shower floor and bathtub
- Bath mat
- Safety rails
- Chair or stool in the shower or bath tub
- Tray with soap, washcloth, long handled bath brush, sponge, or mitt as needed within reach
- Shower cap

- Large bath towel
- Bath thermometer
- Lubricating preparations for water or to apply after bath
- Oatmeal, cornstarch, baking soda for medicated bath
- Talcum powder

Resident

- Explain purpose of procedure and expected results
- Provide privacy during the bath or shower with curtain, screen, and closed door

❧ INTERVENTIONS

1. Perform handwashing.
2. Become familiar with type and pattern of bathing, assistance or aids needed, skin condition, presence of dressings or casts.

3. Cleanse, disinfect, and rinse the bathtub, place a rubber mat on the floor of the shower or in the tub if skid-proof strips are not present.

4. Run water in the tub to half full and test the temperature with the thermometer to obtain a range of 98-104°F or run water into the shower and test on the inner arm for a comfortable temperature.

5. Add medications or other agents to tub water if medicated bath is given.

6. Assist to stand in the shower, or sit on a stool or chair in the shower or tub, inform the resident of the use of the rails for support in getting in and out to prevent falls.

7. Remain with the resident if weak or assistance is needed in washing.

8. Limit the tub bath to less than 15 minutes and shower to less than 10 minutes depending on fatigue and weakness status, check frequently for hypotension if receiving antihypertensive medications.

9. Assist out of the tub or shower, wrap in the bath towel, allow to sit on a chair, and assist to dry if needed, especially in the skin folds.

10. Apply lubricating oil or lotion, talcum powder according to preference and skin condition.

11. Assist to dress if needed or supply aids for dressing independently (see Dressing/Personal Grooming).

12. Clean, disinfect, and rinse tub or shower floor and shower chair after use.

❧ PROBLEM-SOLVING ACTIONS

1. Transport resident to the tub room via a shower chair if unable to walk the distance without fatigue.

2. Place a call light within reach for resident to call for assistance; remain with resident if weak and remove from bath or shower if complaining of weakness or faintness.

3. Prevent intrusion and protect privacy by hanging an "In Use" sign on the door.

4. Protect from drafts and chilling during bathing.

5. Encourage independence in the bathing procedure by supplying aids such as long-handled brush, hand mitt, liquid soap, stools, and hand rails.

6. Inform the resident to refrain from adjusting or adding water as this could result in burns.

❧ EVALUATION

Improved comfort and cleanliness by bathing; skin intact and free from soil, odor, dryness, pruritus

BED, OCCUPIED

aking an occupied bed involves the changing of linens with an individual in bed to provide a clean and comfortable environment and prevent skin irritation and possible impairment. It is done following a bedbath or when the bed becomes soiled or wet. It requires the movement of the individual in bed and can be performed from one side to another or from top to bottom if the bed must remain in Fowler's position for circulatory or respiratory conditions. More than one person may be needed to make an occupied bed to conserve the resident's energy and assist in lifting or supporting activities.

ASSESSMENT

Ability to lie flat in bed and move in bed independently, bedrest status, energy and activity tolerance level

NURSING DIAGNOSES

High Risk for Impaired Skin Integrity; Fatigue; Activity Intolerance

GOAL

Clean, comfortable, wrinkle-free bed changed daily or when needed

INTERVENTIONS

Equipment/Supplies

- Flat sheets (2) or a flat sheet and contour sheet
- Mattress pad
- Pillow cases
- Draw sheet
- Bedspread
- Blanket

- Comfort device (sheepskin)
- Bed protectors
- Bath blanket
- Disposable gloves
- Laundry bag or hamper

Resident

- Explain purpose of procedure and expected results
- Place in sidelying position and change side as needed; place as close to the edge of the bed as possible

PROCEDURE

1. Perform handwashing.
2. Lock the bed and raise to working height.
3. Lower the side rail on the working side of the bed.
4. Loosen top linens and grasp the center of the bedspread with both hands and fold over to the bottom of the bed; fold and place on the back of a chair if it is to be reused or place in laundry bag.

5. Place the bath blanket over the top sheet and, while holding the top in place with one hand, pull the sheet down to the foot of the bed in gathers and remove, fold and place on the back of the chair if it is to be reused for the bottom sheet or discard in the laundry bag.

6. Move the mattress to the top of the bed by grasping the sides and sliding upward with the assistance of another person on the other side or have the resident pull upward at the head of the bed.

7. Remove the call light, TV control or other attachments on the lower sheet.

8. Move the resident to the far side of the bed in supine or sidelying position and allow to hold onto the side rail if able.

9. Remove the pillow and take off the pillow case and discard in laundry bag, place pillow on a clean area; the pillow can be left in place for head support.

10. Loosen the top and side of the bottom sheet and draw sheet, if used, and roll the soiled linen towards the center of the bed to rest up against the resident.

11. Smooth the mattress pad to remove the wrinkles and place the unfolded clean or folded top sheet on the bed.

12. Unfold and center the sheet on the side of the bed with the hem placed in line with the bottom of the mattress (should not be tucked in at the bottom).

13. Lift head of mattress with the nondominant hand and tuck the sheet under the mattress.

14. Make a mitered corner by forming a triangle at the corner, tucking in the lower portion, holding it against the mattress and folding the triangular part down over the hand and tucking under the mattress.

15. Tuck the remaining part of the sheet at the side under the mattress moving downward to the foot of the bed.

16. Raise the side rail and reposition to the opposite side of the bed over the rolled soiled sheet onto the clean sheet.

17. Lower the side rail on the opposite side and loosen the bottom linens, roll the soiled linens to the edge of the bed and discard in the laundry bag.

18. Smooth the mattress pad, unroll the clean sheet and drawsheet, if used, and pull taut to remove wrinkles; place bed protector under the buttocks if used.

19. Proceed at the top to tuck in the sheet and make a mitered corner, tuck in the side under the mattress as for the other side.

20. Reposition to the center of the bed and replace the pillow case with a clean one if it was removed; fold pillow lengthwise and slip into clean case.

21. Place the top sheet on the bath blanket and center with the hem at the head of the bed; unfold to the foot of the bed and open allowing the sides to hang over the bed.

22. Place the blanket and bedspread over the top sheet allowing about 6 inches of the top of the sheet to be folded over them.

23. Hold the top linens and reach under them with the other hand to remove the bath blanket.

24. Tuck the top linens under the mattress at the foot of the bed and make mitered corners.

25. Make a toe pleat by grasping the top linens and lifting to form a pleat and allowing for space to move the feet.

26. Provide extra pillows and elevate head of bed as needed, raise side rails, lower bed, and replace call light and other attachments to the sheet.

27. Remove bag of soiled linen and place in laundry hamper.

❧ PROBLEM SOLVING ACTIONS

1. Resident should be protected from all seams in the linen by placing the bottom sheet with the right side up and top sheet with the right side down.

2. Fitted bottom sheet can be used if available to prevent the sheet from being pulled out.

3. A turning sheet can be used to change the position without pulling or pushing the resident which can cause skin damage.

4. Avoid allowing the soiled linens to touch staff's clothing.

5. Protect clean linens by plastic or other covering.

❧ EVALUATION

Linen change with resident in bed; clean, wrinkle-free with no evidence of dampness or debris

BED, UNOCCUPIED

*M*aking an unoccupied bed involves the changing of linens in an empty bed with the top linens either folded down or brought up to the top of the bed, especially if the resident is up all day. Frequency of linen change depends on individual needs, and the amount of time spent in bed.

ASSESSMENT

Amount of time in bed, extent of soiling of the linens, amount and type of linen that needs to be changed

NURSING DIAGNOSES

High Risk for Impaired Skin Integrity; Sleep Pattern Disturbance

GOAL

Clean, comfortable wrinkle free bed

INTERVENTIONS

Equipment/Supplies

- Flat sheets (2) or a flat sheet and contour sheet
- Mattress pad
- Pillow cases
- Bedspread
- Blanket
- Bed protectors
- Disposable gloves
- Laundry bag or hamper

Resident

- Explain purpose of procedure and expected results

PROCEDURE

1. Perform handwashing.
2. Raise bed to working height, put in a flat position and lower side rails.
3. Remove pillows and take cases off and place in laundry bag.
4. Loosen all the linen on both sides starting at the head of the bed.
5. Grasp the bedspread at the top and fold and pull it to the bottom, remove and place on the back of a chair.
6. Remove the top sheet the same way if it is to be used as a bottom sheet or roll up and place in the laundry bag if soiled.
7. Grasp the bottom sheet and roll downward and place in the laundry bag.
8. Grasp side of the mattress and move upward to the head of the bed.
9. Perform handwashing before handling the clean linens.
10. Smooth mattress pad to remove wrinkles.

11. Place clean bottom sheet or folded top sheet on half of the bed, unfold, and center with the seam in line with the lower edge of the mattress.

12. Lift mattress at the top with the nondominant hand and tuck the sheet under the mattress.

13. Make a mitered corner by lifting the side edge of the sheet and holding at a right angle, tucking the hanging bottom edge under the mattress, dropping the top and tucking it under the mattress.

14. Tuck the rest of the sheet under the mattress moving toward the foot of the bed.

15. Place the top sheet and blanket on the bed and center and unfold on the same side of the bed with the top edge of the sheet in line with the top of the mattress and the top edge of the blanket about 6 inches lower.

16. Tuck in the top layers at the bottom of the mattress and make a mitered corner; do not tuck in the sides but fold the top of the sheet over the blanket at the top of the bed.

17. Move to the other side and repeat the same procedure for the bottom and top linens; pull the bottom sheet taut and smooth before tucking under the mattress.

18. Place bed protectors on the bottom sheet if needed.

19. Make a toe pleat by grasping the top linens with both hands and pulling upward and fold backward into a pleat to allow for space to move feet.

20. Fanfold top linens downward to the halfway point on the bed.

21. Put on clean pillow cases by laying the open case on the bed, folding the pillow lengthwise and holding it under the arm, sliding the pillow into the case held open by the other hand; adjust the corners and place at the head of the bed.

22. Lower bed, replace call light and other attachments.

23. Remove laundry bag of soiled linen and place in laundry hamper.

❧ PROBLEM-SOLVING ACTIONS

1. Resident should be protected from all seams in the linen by placing the bottom sheet with right side up and the top sheet with right side down.

2. Fitted bottom sheet can be used if available.

3. Avoid allowing soiled linens to touch staff's clothing, wear gloves if the linens are soiled with blood or body fluids.

4. Protect clean linens by plastic or other covering.

5. When linens are removed, they should be observed for dentures, other prostheses, or valuables to prevent loss of personal belongings.

6. Linen change can be performed daily, every 2-3 days, or even every week depending on individual need.

7. The top linen is left at the top of the mattress instead of fanfolded downward for a closed bed.

❧ EVALUATION

Linen changed and maintained in clean, wrinkle free state

BEDBATH, COMPLETE

The complete bedbath is performed for those on bedrest who need total or partial assistive care. It is done to cleanse the skin to remove soil, dead epithelial cells, microorganisms, and promote comfort, exercise, and relaxation. The aging skin becomes thinner, drier, and more fragile and requires special considerations in regard to soaps, oils, and frequency of bathing. Based on bedrest status, ability for movement in bed, skin integrity, and general condition, a complete bedbath can be performed daily or alternated with a partial bedbath. While the complete bedbath involves the cleansing of all body parts, the partial bedbath involves the cleansing of the face, hands, axillae, back, and genital/anal areas, and an evening procedure involves cleansing of the face and hands. A variety of modifications can be made to perform this procedure depending on the ability of the individual to participate and the availability of assistive aids. The bath can be performed completely by the staff, or set up for the individual to wash the face, arms, chest, and perineal area or as much of the bath as one is able to perform without fatigue or other adverse effects. In either case, medical asepsis dictates that the order of bathing starts at the cleanest part (the face) and moves down the body to the least clean parts, terminating with the genital/anal areas. Other procedures that provide cleanliness and comfort can also be performed before, during, or after the bath (see Backrub, Oral/Teeth Management, Dentures, Nail Management, Perineal Management, Shaving, Electric/Safety Razors).

❧ ASSESSMENT

Skin condition (color, texture, pigmentation, erythema, edema, temperature, dryness, lesions, odors) skin sensitivities, preference of toilet articles, preference for time of day and frequency/type of bath, ability for self-care

❧ NURSING DIAGNOSES

Activity Intolerance, Self-Care Deficit, Bathing/Hygiene; High Risk of Impaired Skin Integrity

❧ GOAL

Maintenance of skin cleanliness, comfort and integrity

❧ INTERVENTIONS

Equipment/Supplies

- Bath basin with water
- Washcloth, bath mitt, sponge
- Bath blanket
- Soap, liquid or bar
- Body lotion, talcum powder
- Bath oil or other moisturizer
- Deodorant
- Disposable gloves, for perineal care

Resident

- Explain purpose of procedure and expected results
- Place in supine position and change position to sidelying as appropriate to reach areas

❧ PROCEDURE

1. Perform handwashing.

2. Become familiar with type and frequency of bathing, assistance and aids needed, special skin needs.

3. Prepare water in the basin at 96-98° F (warm) or 98-104° F (hot) depending on the condition of the skin and place all articles within reach at the bedside.

4. Adjust the room temperature and remove any drafts that can cause chilling.

5. Provide a bedpan or urinal if needed.

6. Remove the top linens without shaking and discard in the linen bag or fold for use as a bottom sheet replacement.

7. Cover with the bath blanket and remove garments, and elastic hose if present.

8. Place as near to side of the bed as possible.

9. Place a towel over the chest and clean the eyes with the damp washcloth moving from the inner to outer canthus, form a mitt with the washcloth and wash the face with water using a finger to wash inside and outside of ears (soap can be used), rinse and pat dry.

10. Place the towel lengthwise under each arm and wash and rinse arms from axillae to the hands, the basin of water can be placed on the towel and the hand immersed to wash and rinse; pat dry following the rinsing.

11. Apply deodorant if desired.

12. Place a towel over the chest and wash, rinse, and pat dry; cover with bath blanket.

13. Place a towel over the abdomen and wash, rinse and pat dry; cover with bath blanket.

14. Place towels lengthwise under each leg and wash, rinse and pat dry; place the basin of water on the towel and immerse each foot and wash, rinse, and pat dry.

15. Change water to continue bath.

16. Position on side and place towel lengthwise under the back and wash, rinse, and pat dry the back and buttocks area.

17. Perfom backrub procedure (see Backrub).

18. Perform perineal care procedure (see Perineal Management).

19. Remove, cleanse, disinfect reusable supplies and store for future use, discard used linens and articles.

20. Replace gown or pajamas with clean garments and proceed with bedmaking procedure.

❧ PROBLEM-SOLVING ACTIONS

1. Using long, firm but gentle strokes in washing, rinsing and drying, is more comfortable for the resident.

2. If rinsing is not thorough, dryness and pruritis will result.

3. Placing the feet and hands in the basin of water softens the nails for easier nail management if done as part of the bath.

4. Warm water temperature should be used for dryer skin, hot water should be tested with a thermometer on the skin of the inner aspect of the forearm and used with caution to prevent burns.

5. Water should be changed any time that it becomes soapy.

6. The washcloth can be folded around the hand to form a mitt which prevents the ends of the cloth from dripping water.

7. Powder should be used sparingly.

8. Range of motion (ROM) should be done during the bath.

9. Allow for as much independence as possible in bathing by setting up all supplies within reach, raising the head of the bed to a tolerable level, and allowing resident to wash as much as able; offer assistance when needed.

10. Perform skin assessment for tissue changes during bath and note and record abnormalities.

11. Utilize principles of body alignment when positioning the resident during the bath and associated procedures.

❧ EVALUATION

Skin intact, clean and free of dryness, irritation, or pruritis; comfort and feeling of well-being maintained

DENTURES

Dentures are removable artificial teeth usually made of plastic that can be complete upper and/or lower, or partial. Denture care is a part of oral care that includes the removal, reinsertion, cleansing and storage of the prostheses. It is done to remove the soft plaque, food deposits, and microorganisms that accumulate on the dentures in order to promote comfort and cleanliness of the mouth and prevent unpleasant odors. In most cases, the removal and insertion of the dentures is performed by the resident, unless a disability prevents this independent activity. Any one of the denture procedures can be completely or partially done by the nurse depending on individual needs. Dentures are removed from unconscious individuals to prevent airway obstruction in the event that they become dislodged. The procedures are performed using medical asepsis techniques.

❧ ASSESSMENT

Type and fit of dentures, redness, irritation, pain or bleeding of gums, ability or need for assistance in caring for and using dentures

❧ NURSING DIAGNOSES

Altered Oral Mucous Membrane; Self-Care Deficit, Hygiene; Pain; High Risk for Infection

❧ GOALS

Daily or more frequent denture care maintained; oral mucous membranes intact and free from discomfort

❧ INTERVENTIONS

Equipment/Supplies

- Covered denture cup containing water
- Mouthwash
- Toothbrush or denture brush
- Nonabrasive dentifrice or tablet for soaking dentures
- Disposable gloves
- Emesis basin
- Denture adhesive or liner
- Tissues, hand towel

Resident

- Explain purpose of procedure and expected results
- Place in semi-Fowler's or sitting position

❧ PROCEDURE

1. Perform handwashing.
2. Become familiar with usual pattern of care, amount of assistance needed, any problems with denture fit that affect chewing, eating or oral tissue integrity.
3. Prepare the container with water and/or soaking tablet and brush with a cleansing agent.
4. Place the towel on the chest under the chin.

5. For denture removal:
   a. Put on disposable gloves.
   b. Cover the thumb and forefinger of the dominant hand with tissue and retract the lip from the denture with the fingers of the nondominant hand, grasp the front of the upper (maxillary) denture with the tissue covered fingers and move up and down to break the seal that provides the vacuum that holds it in place, slide it out of the mouth and place it in the denture cup of water with denture cleanser.
   c. Grasp the lower (mandibular) denture with the tissue covered fingers and lift it up and out of the mouth and place it in the same denture cup.
   d. If partial denture is present, grasp both sides of the denture where it meets the natural teeth and exert an even pressure to lift it out of its position in the mouth and place in the denture cup of water with denture cleanser.
   e. Allow rinsing of the mouth with diluted mouthwash after removal.
   f. Cleanse the gingiva with a soft brush or sponge-tip applicator with strokes from the front to back and assess for irritated or sore areas.

6. For denture cleansing:
   a. Place the emesis basin in the sink and line with a washcloth to prevent damage to the dentures if they are dropped.
   b. Hold the dentures firmly over the emesis basin, wet under running warm water, and brush all areas with a dentifrice, preferably a powder.
   c. Hold firmly under warm running water and rinse well.
   d. Store in a labeled, clean, covered denture cup containing water for overnight or when not in use.

7. For denture insertion:
   a. Apply denture paste or liner.
   b. Moisten dentures with water to facilitate insertion.
   c. Grasp upper plate with fingers on dominant hand and insert, press against gums to secure in place.
   d. Grasp lower plate and gently rotate to place in the mouth and gently press against gums.

8. Wipe mouth with towel, remove gloves and discard with other used articles.

9. Cleanse and rinse reusable articles and store in clean container or plastic bag.

PROBLEM-SOLVING ACTIONS

1. Loose dentures can fall out and become lost in linens or other areas.

2. Store dentures in warm water as hot water can warp or change the shape, thus affecting the fit.

3. If paste dentifrice is difficult to remove, use powder type.

4. Cleansing agents that scratch dentures can cause tissue irritation.

5. Note any difficulty with chewing or eating, chips or rough areas on dentures, poor fit of dentures and refer to a dentist for correction.

6. Encourage as much independence in denture care procedures as abilities allow, especially in removing and inserting the prostheses.

EVALUATION

General condition and comfort of oral mucous membrane and dentures; dentures in place for eating, speaking and during the waking hours

DRESSING AND PERSONAL GROOMING

Dressing and personal grooming is the provision of clothing and cosmetics or other articles such as jewelry that enhance personal appearance and self-esteem. It also includes assistive devices that encourage an individual to perform self care activities with independence or minimal assistance. Specific procedures that are part of grooming for reference are Hair, Grooming/Shampoo, and Shaving, Electric/Safety Razors. Attention to dressing and grooming needs is given daily.

ASSESSMENT

Activity status and ability to perform self care, preferences in dress and grooming

NURSING DIAGNOSES

Self-Esteem Disturbance; Self-Care Deficit, Dressing/Grooming

GOAL

Maximal participation in daily dressing and grooming routine

INTERVENTIONS

Equipment/Supplies

- Cosmetics in a container within reach on a table with a mirror on a stand

- Articles of clean clothing

- Devices appropriate to individual needs, long or built-up handles on articles, suction cups or wall mounting to hold

Resident

- Position of comfort with articles in position for use, usually sitting to avoid the need to bend over

PROCEDURE

1. Perform handwashing.
2. Become familiar with ability and interest in self care, type of clothing and devices needed.
3. Provide clothing that is easy to care for, loose fitting, front closures with zippers or velcro, elastic waists and cuffs, slacks or jumpers, slip on shoes with velcro closures.
4. Provide devices such as button hooks, zipper pulls, dressing stick with hooks, stocking or sock with long handles for pulling on, mirror that stands, mounted on wall, or that can be hung around neck.
5. Slip weaker limb into clothing first and then the stronger, hook or close articles of clothing in front and shift around to the back, leave a necktie tied and slip over head and tighten.
6. Prepare the articles in order of dressing or applying cosmetics, give partial assistance when needed while encouraging and supporting efforts at self care.
7. Provide laundry services to ensure clean clothing.
8. Allow resident to comment on feelings about appearance.

PROBLEM-SOLVING ACTIONS

1. Additional assistive devices can be utilized for those with loss of limbs, mental or sensory deprivation, and neuromuscular disorders.

2. Store articles within reach to avoid need for reaching or stooping, color code or label drawers and closets for easier identification of storage places.

3. Integrate physical and occupational therapy regimens with dressing and grooming activities.

4. Comfortable and appropriate underwear should be worn under clothing; gowns should not be left on under clothing.

5. Clothing should not be put on backwards.

6. Non-skid footwear should be used and those who stand, transfer, or ambulate should wear shoes and stockings.

EVALUATION

Maximal independence in dressing and grooming activities; neat, clean appearance

EYE GLASSES AND CONTACT LENSES

Eye glasses and contact lenses are visual aids prescribed and worn to enhance visual acuity. Eye glass frames are made of metal or plastic, as are eye glass lenses. Contact lenses are made of soft or hard plastic. They are thin curved disks with soft lenses covering the entire cornea and molding to eye shape, or hard lenses covering part of the cornea and touching the eye during blinking. The contact lenses are small, easily lost, and improper handling can cause damage or injury to the eye. The procedures included in the care of eye glasses are cleaning and storing; and in the care of contact lenses, removal, handling, cleansing, inserting, and storing. Usually, the resident performs these procedures but may require assistance by the nurse if illness or disability prevents independence.

ASSESSMENT

Visual acuity with and without glasses or contact lenses, type of visual aid and purpose, ability to perform care procedures, fit and irritation of skin on nose or ears from glasses, redness, irritation, pain in eyes from contact lenses

NURSING DIAGNOSES

Sensory/Perceptual Alterations (Visual); High Risk for Impaired Skin or Tissue Integrity; High Risk for Infection

GOALS

Maintenance of visual acuity with care and use of visual aid; skin and mucous membrane integrity preserved

INTERVENTIONS

Equipment/Supplies

- Eye glass case or lens container with label for right and left lenses
- Cleansing and rinsing solution or normal saline for contact lenses in a small container
- Wetting, soaking, and disinfecting solution for contact lenses in a small container

- Cleansing solution or commercial wipes for eye glasses
- Small soft cloth or paper towel

Resident

- Explain purpose of procedure and expected results
- Place in position of comfort

PROCEDURE

1. Perform handwashing.
2. Become familiar with the type of visual aid, if worn continuously or for specific purposes such as reading.

3. Clean eye glasses with warm soapy water and dry with a soft lint-free cloth or paper; apply by fitting the nose piece over the bridge of the nose and the two arms up and around the upper part of the ear, remove and place in an eye glass case with the arms folded down when not in use and store in a drawer.

4. To remove hard contact lenses, separate the eyelids with the thumb and finger of the dominant hand and stretch towards the temporal side, then move the lids together to break the suction, catch the lens in the other hand, and place in the case containing the soaking solution in the right and left sections, respectively.

5. To remove soft lenses, raise the upper eyelids and hold in position with the non-dominant hand, place the thumb and finger of the dominant hand on the lenses, pinch and catch when it comes off the cornea, and place in the case containing normal saline in the right and left sections, respectively.

6. To clean hard lenses, apply a few drops of cleansing solution on each lens separately to avoid mixing the right and left, rub gently with the fingers to remove any dirt, rinse well with tap water, place in soaking solution or store in the case.

7. To clean soft lenses, apply a few drops of cleansing solution on each lens separately, rub gently with the fingers or in the palm of the hand to remove film and dirt, rinse well with the cleansing solution, place in a disinfectant solution in the appropriate sections of the case and let stand for 4 or more hours and time well with normal saline.

8. Soft lenses can also be cleaned by heat disinfection by applying normal saline solution, gently rubbing and placing in the case in the appropriate sections filled with the saline and then placing the case in an electric disinfecting unit for a specified period of time.

9. To insert hard lenses, wash hands, remove from the case and rinse, wet each lens with solution, place the correct lens for the correct eye on the index finger of the dominant hand with the concave side up and exposed, request the resident to look upward and separate the eyelids with the thumb and finger of the non-dominant hand, then place the lens directly on the cornea.

10. To insert soft lenses, remove from the case and rinse, place the lens between the thumb and finger of the dominant hand with the concave side upward, note edges that point inward for the correct position for insertion; wet with saline and while the resident is requested to look upward, separate the eyelids with the non-dominant hand and gently place the lens on the surface of the cornea.

11. Remove the solution from the containers and case, rinse and air dry for future use.

❧ PROBLEM-SOLVING ACTIONS

1. Careful attention to ensure that the correct lens is applied to the correct eye is essential; small medicine cups that are labeled right and left with tape can be used if a case is not available.

2. If contact lens is off-center, request the resident to look toward the lens and gently push it toward the pupil with the eyelid.

3. Note and report redness, irritation, or pain in the eye while wearing the contact lenses, remove or limit wearing until corrected if possible; if eyes feel or appear dry, instill sterile normal saline before removing contact lenses.

4. Pads can be attached to the part of the glasses that rests on the bridge or sides of the nose and behind the ears if pressure causes redness, soreness, or skin breaks; referral to an optometrist for readjustment of the fit can be made.

5. Notify physician that resident has contact lenses if eye medications are ordered.

6. Prolonged lens retention of some types of contacts can cause corneal damage.

7. Commercially-prepared cleansing tissue wipes are available to clean eye glasses.

❧ EVALUATION

Appropriate and careful care and use of eye glasses or contact lenses demonstrated; no evidence of eye, nose or ear irritation

EYE MANAGEMENT OF THE UNCONSCIOUS RESIDENT

*T*he eye care of those in coma includes procedures that cleanse and lubricate both eyes and
eyelids. It is done to remove the secretions that accumulate when the resident is not able
to blink the eyes or wipe the secretions away. The procedures are performed using medical
asepsis technique.

ASSESSMENT

Dried secretions or crusting causing the eyelids to stick together; redness, exudate from eye infection

NURSING DIAGNOSES

High Risk for Infection, High Risk for Impaired Tissue Integrity; Self-Care Deficit (Hygiene)

GOAL

Complete care of eyes to prevent infection and dryness

INTERVENTIONS

Equipment/Supplies

- Sterile basin with sterile normal saline solution or other ordered solution
- Disposable gloves
- Cotton balls
- Artificial tears, eye ointment
- Gauze eye pads and tape
- Hand towel

Resident

- Place in supine position with head of bed slightly elevated

PROCEDURE

1. Perform handwashing.
2. Become familiar with type of solution and/or ointment ordered and frequency of care, and if done with other personal hygiene care.
3. Place the hand towel over the chest and put on disposable gloves.
4. Prepare the solution in the basin and open the packages of supplies needed and place within reach.
5. Using the cotton balls moistened with the saline or other solution; wipe each eye from the inner to outer canthus, one stroke per cotton ball.
6. Gently dry the eyes with a clean cotton ball.
7. Administer commercially-prepared artificial tears or ointment to provide moisture (see Medications, Eye Drops/Ointment).
8. Place a moist gauze eye pad on the eyes and tape in place.
9. Remove gloves and dispose with other used supplies using Universal Precautions.

❧ PROBLEM-SOLVING ACTIONS

1. Note any inflammation or other eye condition caused by the absence of the corneal reflex in the unconscious resident.

2. If any infection is present in one eye, cleanse the eye free of infection first.

3. Cleansing the right eye first assists in recalling which eye has been cared for if interrupted during the procedure.

4. Always use sterile supplies to prevent eye infection.

❧ EVALUATION

Proper care of the eyes and eyelids demonstrated

EYE PROSTHESIS

An eye prosthesis is a plastic orb made in the shape and appearance of the resident's normal eye. Those who have experienced the surgical removal of an eye (enucleation) related to pathology or trauma can use a prosthesis to preserve body image and self esteem. The procedures included in the care of the eye socket and prosthesis are removal of the prosthesis, cleansing of the prosthesis, irrigation of the eye socket, insertion of the prosthesis, and storage of the prosthesis. In most cases, the procedures are carried out by the resident. In those with paralysis or impaired ability to use the hands and arms or those who are unconscious, the care can be completely or partially done by the nurse depending on individual needs. The procedures are performed using medical asepsis techniques.

ASSESSMENT

Which eye has the prosthesis, ability or need for assistance in caring for prosthesis and eye socket, use of eyeglasses, eye socket irritation, redness, drainage or secretions, crusting

NURSING DIAGNOSES

High Risk for Injury; Body Image Disturbance; Impaired Tissue Integrity

GOAL

Maintenance of eye prosthesis and eye socket tissue for optimal benefit to health and sense of well being

INTERVENTIONS

Equipment/Supplies

- Small basin or covered cup
- Normal saline solution
- Opthalmic solution for irrigation
- Irrigation set (syringe and container)
- Towel and tissues
- Gauze squares or pads
- Suction cup
- Emesis basin
- Disposable gloves

Resident

- Explain purpose of procedure and expected results
- Place in sitting position or in a sidelying position if unconscious

PROCEDURE

1. Perform handwashing.
2. Become familiar with usual pattern of prosthesis and eye socket care, which eye has the prosthesis, independence or amount of assistance needed.
3. Place the towel or a protective waterproof protector over the chest and shoulders.
4. Place a gauze square at the bottom of the covered container to prevent damage to the prosthesis during storage and fill with saline or water.
5. Put on gloves and gently wipe the eye from the inner to outer canthus with a gauze square and saline or ophthalmic solution.

6. Squeeze the suction cup and remove prosthesis by placing the suction cup (after squeezing) at the center of the prosthesis and, while gently pulling down on the lower eye lid, pull the prosthesis downward and upward under the upper lid and out of the socket; catch in a hand if a suction cup is not used.

7. Wash the prosthesis with water or ophthalmic solution and place it on the gauze in the covered cup of solution.

8. Irrigate the socket with ophthalmic solution directing the syringe from the inner to outer canthus allowing the solution to drain into an emesis basin held by the resident or propped in place; cleanse any crusts from the eye lids with gauze and solution and pat the eye dry.

9. To insert the prosthesis, squeeze the suction cup and place on the center of the moist prosthesis or hold it between the thumb and finger; gently pull the upper lid upward with the other hand and slip the upper part of the prosthesis under the upper lid and then gently pull downward on the lower lid and slip the lower part of the prosthesis under the lower lid; remove the suction cup if used.

10. Note that the prosthesis is in proper position in the socket.

11. Store the prosthesis in the covered cup of solution when not in use.

12. Discard used articles and clean and store reusable supplies according to Universal Precautions.

❧ PROBLEM-SOLVING ACTIONS

1. Prosthesis can remain in the eye socket without daily care unless socket becomes irritated, dry, secretions accumulate, or surgery or diagnostic procedures are scheduled.

2. Wearing a pair of glasses with clear plastic lenses can protect the good eye from injury when participating in activities.

3. Avoid cleansing the prosthesis with alcohol, ether, or acetone as these can dull the plastic material.

4. Gentle rubbing over the closed eyelid towards the nose with a finger can alleviate itching of the side with the prosthesis.

❧ EVALUATION

Proper care of prosthesis and eye socket demonstrated

FOOT MANAGEMENT

Foot management is the daily assessment, bathing, lubrication, and protection of the feet. It is done to promote cleanliness and peripheral circulation of the feet. Foot care is especially important in those with Diabetes Mellitus or peripheral circulatory conditions because of their susceptibility to infection and skin breakdown. If required, trimming of the toenails is performed by a podiatrist.

ASSESSMENT

Skin on the feet for blisters, rubbed, cracked, dry, irritated areas, breakdown or injuries, discoloration, tactile sensory perception changes, areas of infection, ingrown toenail, corns, calluses

NURSING DIAGNOSES

High Risk for Impaired Skin Integrity; Sensory Alteration (Tactile), Altered Tissue Perfusion (Peripheral); High Risk for Infection

GOALS

Skin on feet intact and free from odor, infection, irritation, and trauma; daily foot care provided

INTERVENTIONS

Equipment/Supplies

- Basin of warm water, mild soap, soft towel, washcloth
- Lotion, talcum powder

- Emery board, applicators
- Waterproof protector material

Resident

- Explain purpose of procedure and expected results
- Place in sitting position with shoes and hose removed

PROCEDURE

1. Perform handwashing.
2. Become familiar with medical conditions that compromise circulation in the feet and assess for need of nail trimming (to be performed by a podiatrist).
3. Place one foot into the basin of warm water and allow to soak for 5 to 10 minutes; check water temperature to prevent burns.
4. Remove foot and pat dry (including between the toes) as rubbing can damage skin.
5. Change the water and immerse the other foot into the basin to soak; dry.
6. Clean under the nails and around the cuticles with a cotton-tipped applicator.
7. File any rough edges with the emery board.
8. Apply lotion or oil preparation to dry areas; place talcum powder between toes and a folded gauze between toes if pressure or friction is present.
9. Apply hose and shoes unless on bedrest.

10. Remove articles and supplies, clean and store for reuse or discard.

❧ PROBLEM-SOLVING ACTIONS

1. Nail trimming can be done by a podiatrist.

2. In those with medical conditions that impair circulation, clean white socks and properly-fitted shoes are preferable to maintain cleanliness and prevent pressure on the feet; rough areas or seams in the socks or shoes should be eliminated.

3. Daily assessment of the feet should be done when care is given and any breaks, blisters, cracks or other abnormalities should be noted.

4. Avoid heat or cold applications if sensory perception is reduced; walking in bare feet should be avoided.

5. Provide warm socks and extra covers to the feet if they are cold.

6. If corns or calluses are present, a podiatrist should be consulted.

7. Special precautions must be taken if the patient suffers from *Diabetes Mellitus*:
   a. Elevate sheets with bed cradle to prevent ulcerations.
   b. To prevent the heels from touching the bed, use pillows to elevate or use heel protectors.
   c. When cleaning the feet, be sure to clean between the toes, and gently rub dry so no moisture remains.
   d. The resident should never go barefoot; socks provide extra protection.
   e. Adding insoles to shoes can cause problems and should be avoided.
   f. Avoid using heating pads, hot water bottles, or electric heaters to heat the feet; put on socks instead.
   g. Avoid wearing socks for more than two hours at a time. Change shoes every five hours to alternate the pressure put on the feet.
   h. Instruct resident not to sit with legs crossed because it decreases circulation to the feet.
   i. Piling heavy linens on the feet can result in loss of circulation.

❧ EVALUATION

Consistent absence of skin breakdown, infection, or trauma on feet

HAIR, GROOMING/SHAMPOO

Hair care is the removal of soil, oils and microorganisms by cleansing and grooming activities to promote circulation to the hair, a healthy scalp, and improved appearance. It also promotes a sense of comfort and body image. It includes the shampoo and rinsing of the hair, massage of the scalp, and combing, brushing, and arranging of the hair according to preference, structure, and condition. The procedures can be done independently or with assistance as needed, in or out of bed. A visiting beautician is also available. Frequency of the shampoo depends on the condition of the hair, and physician's orders, but grooming is performed daily as part of personal hygiene care.

ASSESSMENT

Type and condition of hair, color, luster, texture and distribution of hair, patterns of care, ability to perform self-care

NURSING DIAGNOSES

Self-Care Deficit, Hygiene/Grooming; Body Image Disturbance

GOAL

Clean, well-groomed hair and general appearance maintained

INTERVENTIONS

Equipment/Supplies

- Tray or trough for the bed
- Waterproof bed protectors
- Receptacle to receive the water on a chair beside the bed
- Two pitchers of warm water
- Bath thermometer
- Two bath towels
- Disposable gloves

- Liquid shampoo, hair conditioner
- Dry shampoo if appropriate
- Portable hair dryer

- Comb with wide, dull pointed teeth
- Brush or pick comb
- Hair lotion or jelly preparation
- Hairpins, barrette, rubber band

Resident

- Explain purpose of procedure and expected results
- Place as close to side of the bed as possible in supine position or sitting in a chair at the sink

PROCEDURE

1. Perform handwashing.
2. Become familiar with type of hair needs and pattern of care, ability to groom own hair and sit at sink for shampoo, availability of salon for hair care.
3. Prepare articles at the bedside for a bed shampoo.
4. Fold top covers down and cover with a bath blanket, place a towel over chest and shoulders.

5. Remove pillow and cover bed with protective sheet.

6. Place the shampoo tray under the head with the body in a slightly diagonal position, drape the trough into the pail on the chair.

7. Check temperature of water in the pitchers (96-104°F).

8. Slowly pour a small amount of water over the hair to dampen, place a washcloth over the eyes to protect from the water and shampoo.

9. Spread the shampoo over all the hair and massage all areas with the pads of the fingers to create a lather and cleanse.

10. Move head to reach all areas during the massaging and add water when needed to maintain the lather.

11. After massage, pour water over the hair to rinse well while stroking the hair with the fingers of the nondominant hand.

12. Repeat the shampoo if a second soaping is needed.

13. Apply a hair conditioner, rinse again, squeeze excess water from the hair and wrap the towel around the head.

14. Dry face, neck, ears with other towel.

15. Remove the tray and other articles from the bed.

16. Rub the hair dry or use an electric hair dryer to blow dry.

17. Comb hair in sections, careful not to pull too harshly to remove snags.

18. Place a clean towel over the shoulders, brush, style, braid, pull back and secure with barrette or band as preferred or requested.

19. Remove gloves and discard with all disposable used supplies, clean, dry and store the reusable equipment.

❧ PROBLEM-SOLVING ACTIONS

1. An improvised tray can be made by forming a rimmed surface using a bath blanket and lining it with plastic to create a waterproofed, shallow device to collect and drain the water from the bed shampoo.

2. Dry shampoos that do not need rinsing can be used to remove soil when a shampoo is not possible.

3. Shampoo at the sink can be performed using a tray over the sink with the neck resting on the tray or resting the head on the edge of the sink, a hose attached to the tap or an irrigating bag can be used to provide the water needed.

4. A shampoo can be performed in the shower if the resident is able to stand long enough for the procedure; a shower chair can be used.

5. Unnecessary exposure to drafts during the shampoo should be avoided to prevent chilling.

6. Hair of the black resident requires special care before and after shampooing such as special shampoos and conditioners or oils and use of a wide-toothed comb or pick to style according to resident preference.

7. Tangled hair should be treated with oil before combing; matting or tangles cannot be cut without written permission.

8. Allow for independence in hair shampoo and grooming by providing all supplies within reach, a mirror, long handles for grooming aids, clip on or velcro curlers, spouted bottle for shampoo, other modifications and instruction in their use.

❧ EVALUATION

Hair that is clean, neat and free from odor, attractively styled

HEARING AIDS

Hearing aids are electronic devices that enhance auditory perception when hearing is impaired. A hearing aid consists of a microphone that receives sound and converts it into energy form, an amplifier that magnifies this energy form, and a receiver that converts the magnified energy into sound and transmits it into the ear. A commonly available hearing aid is one that fits over and behind the ear with a small case containing the components and an earmold, connected to each other by a small tube. This type can also be attached to an eyeglass arm. Another type is a small device containing all the components that is molded to fit the ear and hardly noticeable when in place. Another type is the body hearing aid, usually reserved for the most severe hearing loss. It includes a device containing all the components attached to or placed in a pocket, undershirt, or harness hung around the neck and an electric cord connecting this device to an earmold that is placed into the ear. The procedures included in the care of a hearing aid are battery change, removal of the earmold, insertion of the earmold, and storage of the device. Usually, the resident performs the procedures involved in the care and use of the hearing aid. Assistance is given to those with impaired abilities and assessment for proper function of the aid is to ensure that hearing is optimal.

❧ ASSESSMENT

Type of aid used, ability to care for the aid or need for assistance, auditory acuity with and without the aid, fit and comfort of aid, ear condition for pain, redness, drainage, swelling

❧ NURSING DIAGNOSES

Sensory/Perceptual Alterations (Auditory); High Risk for Impaired Skin Integrity; Body Image Disturbance

❧ GOAL

Maintenance of hearing aid use for optimal benefit to health and sense of well-being

❧ INTERVENTIONS

Equipment/Supplies

- Hearing aid and associated parts
- Battery if appropriate
- Toothpicks or pipe cleaners
- Small basin of warm, soapy water
- Soft cloth hand towel or paper towel
- Case or container to store hearing aid

Resident

- Explain purpose of procedure and expected results
- Place in sitting or position of comfort

❧ PROCEDURE

1. Perform handwashing.
2. Become familiar with the usual pattern of hearing aid care, amount of assistance needed to perform use and care procedures.
3. Turn the hearing aid off and volume completely down depending on type of device.

4. Remove the earmold by rotating forward and pulling it out with the dominant hand.

5. Unclip the earmold from the case containing the components of the hearing aid.

6. Wash the earmold with warm, soapy water, rinse and dry; the ear-mold can be immersed in the soapy water if it is not permanently connected to the receiver or case; those connected to a case or the ear-mold should be wiped with a damp cloth and not washed with or immersed in soapy water.

7. Use a toothpick or pipe cleaner to remove any debris or cerumen being careful not to push this into the earmold opening.

8. Store the hearing aid in its case and place in a drawer when not in use after removal and cleansing to prevent damage or misplacement.

9. Reinsert the earmold in the right or left ear as appropriate by lining up the parts with the ear and inserting the canal part and then rotating the earmold backwards into the ear, position the tube and case over the ear or the case and wire on the garment and adjust to resident's preference; the in-the-ear earmold fits flush with the ear canal and needs no further adjustments.

10. Turn the hearing aid on and adjust the volume.

11. Remove and dispose of used articles and clean and store reusable supplies.

❧ PROBLEM-SOLVING ACTIONS

1. Battery should be checked periodically and replaced when necessary; when the hearing aid is not in use, the battery should be removed and stored separately.

2. Avoid any exposure to heat and humidity as this can change the shape of the plastic device and affect the fit.

3. If sound is weak, whistling, or absent, check the battery, make sure the volume is turned on, that all connections are secure, and for improper insertion of the battery and earmold.

4. Refer to an audiologist if hearing acuity has changed. Check operating manual to troubleshoot problems, or contact the hearing aid dealer.

5. The ear should be washed and dried daily, avoid using cotton-tipped applicator to cleanse the ear canal.

❧ EVALUATION

Proper care and use of hearing aid demonstrated

NAIL MANAGEMENT

N*ail management is the regular care of the toenails and fingernails to promote cleanliness,*
and skin integrity of tissues, to prevent infection, and injury from scratching by fingernails
or pressure of shoes on toenails. It includes cleansing, trimming, smoothing, and cuticle care
and is usually done during the bath. Nails can become thinner and more brittle in the elderly
and thicker if peripheral circulation is impaired. Nails are also important in assessment, as
changes occur with certain medical conditions, such as, clubbing with chronic obstructive
pulmonary disease or cardiac disease, color change with circulatory or lymphatic impairment
and certain drug therapy. Common to the elderly are ingrown nails and fungal infections of
the toenails; dry, brittle, ridges, and thickening of all nails. Nail care, especially trimming, is
performed by a podiatrist in those with diabetes mellitus and peripheral vascular disease.

ASSESSMENT

General condition of the nails, color, texture, length, dryness, cleanliness, redness and swelling at
cuticles, impaired peripheral circulation (peripheral pulse, slow growth, color)

NURSING DIAGNOSES

High Risk for Infection; Altered Tissue Perfusion (Peripheral); High Risk for Impaired Tissue Integrity

GOALS

Maintain nail management for optimal comfort, appearance, and integrity

INTERVENTIONS

Equipment/Supplies

- Nail clipper
- Orange sticks
- Emery boards
- Nail brush

- Lotion
- Basin of warm soapy water
- 2 towels

Resident

- Explain purpose of procedure and
  expected results

PROCEDURE

1. Perform handwashing.
2. Immerse hands or feet in a basin of warm soapy water to cleanse and soften the nails for ease in
   cleansing and trimming; use a soft brush if necessary to cleanse under and around the nails.
3. Remove debris from under the nails with an orange stick while soaking.
4. Remove the hands or feet from the basin and pat dry.
5. Apply lotion and massage into the cuticles and push back with a towel; avoid cutting any cuticle.
6. Trim the nails with a clipper, straight across for the toenails, rounded for the fingernails.
7. Smooth the nails with an emery board.

8. Apply hose and shoes or slippers as appropriate.
9. Discard removed nails, cleanse basin and articles used and store for future use.

❧ PROBLEM-SOLVING ACTIONS

1. Nails that are ingrown, thickened, or infected should be cared for by a podiatrist.
2. Cutting should not be any shorter than at the line even with the nail folds on each side.
3. It is usually necessary to obtain permission from the resident to cut the nails.
4. When performed at bath time, the nail care can be done following the procedure or as a separate procedure when needed at the convenience of the resident.

❧ EVALUATION

Nails and surrounding skin care performed safely and correctly; absence of abnormal nail conditions such as ingrown nails and infections

ORAL /TEETH MANAGEMENT

O ral and teeth care is the removal of soft plaque and food particles, bacteria, and odors to promote physical and psychological comfort. It prevents dental cavities and abnormal mouth conditions that result from medications or disease. It includes procedures such as brushing and flossing, gum massage, and mouth rinsing. It is performed in the morning, at bedtime, and after meals depending on individual needs. The procedures can be done independently or with assistance in those with impaired ability to use the hands and arms.

ASSESSMENT

Presence of partial dentures, saliva production, bleeding, lesions, or sore oral mucosa, alterations in taste, mouth breathing, medication regimen, ability to perform own care

NURSING DIAGNOSES

High Risk for Infection, Altered Oral Mucous Membrane; Self-Care Deficit, Hygiene; Sensory/ Perceptual Alterations, Gustatory

GOALS

Oral and teeth care maintained; oral mucous membranes intact and free from discomfort

INTERVENTIONS

Equipment/Supplies

- Toothbrush (electric or manual)
- Dental floss (unwaxed if appropriate)
- Mouthwash
- Dentifrice (paste or powder)
- Cotton-tipped applicators

- Emesis basin
- Water in a glass with drinking straw
- Petroleum jelly or other moisturizer
- Disposable gloves
- Tissues and hand towel

Resident

- Explain purpose of procedure and expected results and benefits
- Place in high-Fowler's position in bed or sitting or standing at sink

PROCEDURE

1. Perform handwashing.
2. Become familiar with the usual pattern of care, preferences in supplies, abnormal mouth or teeth conditions, amount of assistance needed.
3. Prepare the articles within reach at the bedside or sink.
4. Place the hand towel on the chest and under the chin and put on gloves.
5. Place emesis basin under the chin or request resident to hold in place.
6. Apply petroleum jelly or other lubricant to lips.
7. Mix some mouthwash in a glass with water and place a straw in it; allow to rinse mouth to remove any food particles or excess saliva.

8. Gently clean between teeth with floss moving it back and forth against each tooth as close to the gum as possible; use a floss holder if available.

9. Wet the toothbrush with some water and brush the lower and upper teeth with strokes from the gum line upward and downward respectively, then the surfaces of the teeth with a back and forth movement, the tongue and the sides of the buccal cavity; move the head from side to side to reach all areas.

10. Allow to sip the solution or water and expectorate into the emesis basin between the brushing of each part or as needed.

11. Massage the gums if appropriate with a cotton swab saturated with mouthwash solution, a brush or rubber stimulator on a handle.

12. Wipe the mouth with tissues during the procedure.

13. Remove gloves and dispose with used articles, clean and store reusable articles for future use.

✌ PROBLEM-SOLVING ACTIONS

1. Oxygenating agents such as a diluted hydrogen peroxide solution can be substituted as a mouthwash if inflammation of mucous membranes is present.

2. Using about 10 short strokes with gentle pressure over 3 to 4 teeth at a time is more beneficial than brushing a whole section of teeth.

3. Avoid brushing if severe inflammation or lesions are present, use mouthwash instead.

4. If the resident must be flat in bed, position on side with face in view and towel and emesis basin under the chin for the procedures.

5. Provide referral to dentist if tooth pain is reported.

6. Allow for independence in mouth and teeth care by providing all supplies and a mirror, padded or jointed handles, suction cup on articles to be used, easily removable caps on toothpaste and solutions, other modifications, and instruct or assist in their use.

7. Provide mouth rinse following medications that cause drying or possible inflammations (inhalants, oxygen, chemotherapy).

✌ EVALUATION

Mouth and teeth clean and free of odors, pain and breaks or irritation

ORAL MANAGEMENT OF THE UNCONSCIOUS RESIDENT

The oral care of the individual in coma includes procedures that cleanse and lubricate the oral cavity, teeth, gums and lips. It is done to remove accumulations of secretions, microorganisms, and residue on the teeth. It also prevents dryness of the mucous membranes and lips. Because of the altered state of consciousness, the ability to swallow is impaired and fluids can be aspirated into the lungs during the procedure. This requires special preventive measures such as positioning and continuous suctioning of the mouth. The procedures are performed using medical asepsis techniques.

❧ ASSESSMENT

Color, dryness, and breaks in mucous membranes, tongue, and skin on lips, presence of natural teeth or dentures, halitosis and presence of sardes (brown, crusty material)

❧ NURSING DIAGNOSES

High Risk for Aspiration, Altered Oral Mucous Membranes

❧ GOAL

Oral mucous membrane integrity and mouth and teeth cleanliness maintained

❧ INTERVENTIONS

Equipment/Supplies

- Soft toothbrush, toothpaste, dental floss if teeth present
- Mouthwash, hydrogen peroxide solution
- Emesis basin
- Disposable gloves
- Suction machine with soft catheter
- Glycerin swabs, petroleum jelly

- Padded tongue blade, bite block
- Plain tongue blades, cotton-tipped applicators
- Asepto syringe
- Gauze squares
- Hand towel

Resident

- Explain what is being done during the procedure
- Place in a sidelying flat position

❧ PROCEDURE

1. Perform handwashing.
2. Become familiar with condition of mouth, type and frequency of care needed, level of consciousness, and absence of reflexes.
3. Place the hand towel and emesis basin under the face and chin, turn head to the side.
4. Prepare the solutions, articles within reach, and turn on suction.
5. Put on gloves.
6. Apply petroleum jelly to the lips to prevent cracking.

7. Insert gauze covered tongue blade into the side of the mouth between the upper and lower teeth to hold the mouth open and insert the bite block between the teeth on the opposite side.

8. Remove the padded tongue blade and irrigate the mouth with warm solution or dilute mouthwash with an asepto syringe, suction fluid with the catheter inserted in the mouth as needed.

9. Cleanse the oral cavity of debris and sores with covered forceps or a tongue depressor and repeat wiping until free of mucous; use hydrogen peroxide solution as an oxidizing agent.

10. If teeth are present, gently brush the surfaces and the tongue, irrigate with warm solution or dilute mouthwash while suctioning to remove the toothpaste and fluid.

11. Floss the teeth with unwaxed dental floss.

12. Change the position to the other side, insert the bite block on the opposite side and repeat the procedure to care for the other side of the mouth.

13. Remove bite block and wipe lips with hand towel.

14. Apply another thin layer of petroleum jelly.

15. Place in position of comfort.

16. Remove gloves and dispose with other used articles according to Universal Precautions and cleanse reusable supplies and store for further use.

❧ PROBLEM-SOLVING ACTIONS

1. Adjust amount of friction used in cleansing according to tissue sensitivity and integrity.

2. The frequency of the application of moisturizing agents to the mouth and lips depends on whether oxygen is administered or mouth breathing is evident.

3. Perform assessment of oral cavity during the procedure using a tongue blade and penlight.

4. Using gauze squares instead of cotton-tipped applicators allows for removal of a greater amount of debris.

❧ EVALUATION

Oral cavity and lips free of secretion accumulation, odors, breaks in tissues, choking or aspiration prevented

PERINEAL MANAGEMENT

Perineal management is the cleansing of the perineal area that includes the genitalia and rectal areas. It promotes cleanliness and comfort and prevents infection by removing irritating secretions or excretions, microorganisms, and offensive odors. The care should be administered daily during bathing, and more frequently following urinary and/or fecal incontinence or if excessive secretions are present. Besides cleansing by washing and drying, special perineal care procedures can be performed by rinsing the area with an irrigation or by soaking the perineal area by sitting in a sitz bath, usually reserved as post-surgical treatments.

❧ ASSESSMENT

Odors, secretions of perineal area, skin at perineal area for redness, edema, pain, inflammation, continence status

❧ NURSING DIAGNOSES

High Risk for Infection; Diarrhea; Altered Pattern of Urinary Elimination; Bowel Incontinence; High Risk for Impaired Skin Integrity

❧ GOALS

Control of odors and cleanliness of perineal area with daily or more frequent care; perineal skin intact and free from irritation

❧ INTERVENTIONS

Equipment/Supplies

- Basin of warm water, mild soap, 2 soft towels, washcloth
- Bath blanket
- Disposable gloves, washcloths
- Waterproof protective pad
- Lotion, talcum powder, deodorant

Resident

- Explain purpose of procedure and expected results
- Place in dorsal recumbent and sidelying position for females, supine and sidelying for males; drape around exposed perineal area to be cleansed

❧ PROCEDURE

1. Perform handwashing.
2. Ascertain whether the procedure is routine or done for other reasons.
3. Offer the urinal or bedpan prior to the procedure if needed.
4. Ensure privacy and warmth and prevent embarrassment by proper draping with a bath blanket.
5. Place the waterproof protector under the hips.
6. Put on disposable gloves.
7. For female perineal care:
   a. Spread legs apart and flex knees while maintaining a drape over the genitalia.

    b. Using the washcloth and soap, wash the mons pubis, rinse and dry.

    c. Moisten the washcloth with water and soap and separate the labia with the thumb and finger of the nondominant hand and wash down the center of the genitalia from front to back, then down each side of the genitalia from front to back using a different part of the washcloth with water and soap.

    d. Rinse the genitalia with the labia separated and pat dry.

    e. Turn to a sidelying position and wash perineum and anus from front to back and rinse and pat dry.

    f. Apply talcum, ointment if needed.

8. For male perineal care:

    a. Hold the penis upright with the nondominant hand and, using a washcloth with water and soap, wash the penis in a circular motion with the dominant hand starting at the urethral tip and continuing with long strokes while moving down penis shaft, fold washcloth to expose clean areas for washing the shaft after the urethra is washed.

    b. Rinse using the same motions as for washing, pat dry.

    c. If uncircumcised, gently retract the foreskin with the dominant hand and hold in place with the nondominant hand while washing the area in a circular motion, rinse and pat dry and allow the retracted foreskin to return to its normal position.

    d. Wash, rinse, and dry the scrotum starting with the anterior part and then, while raising and holding the scrotum in the palm of the nondominant hand, wash, rinse and dry the rest of the scrotum and perineum.

    e. Turn to the sidelying position and wash, rinse and dry the anal area.

    f. Apply talcum powder or ointment if needed.

9. Change the gown, bed linens if needed.

10. Place in a comfortable position; cleanse and store articles for future use.

❧ PROBLEM-SOLVING ACTIONS

1. If perineal care is given as part of a bedbath, perform this procedure following the washing of other body parts, change water and complete the bath with the back care procedure.

2. Allow the resident to independently perform own perineal care if possible, give assistance if needed.

3. If feces is present on the buttocks or perineal area, remove with tissue, then soap and water using disposable washcloth, before performing perineal care.

4. If performing perineal care on the opposite sex, try to prevent embarrassment and anxiety for the resident; in the case of male residents, a nonchalant attitude can prevent a physically induced erection.

5. Assessment of the genitalia and anal area skin for irritation should be done during perineal care on those who are incontinent of urine and/or feces.

❧ EVALUATION

Comfort, cleanliness and skin integrity maintained with daily perineal care

SHAVING, ELECTRIC/SAFETY RAZORS

Shaving of the male resident can be performed with an electric or safety razor depending on preference and availability of equipment. It is usually done as a part of daily personal hygiene, although every other day is sufficient for some based on the beard growth. It is done to promote cleanliness and a positive body image. Usually, the resident or a visiting barber performs this procedure, but the nurse can shave the resident if illness or disability prevents independence.

ASSESSMENT

Frequency of shaving, type of shaving device used, condition of skin on face (redness, irritation, breaks), blood clotting disorder or anticoagulant therapy

NURSING DIAGNOSES

High Risk for Infection; High Risk for Impaired Skin Integrity

GOAL

Safe removal of facial hair when needed

INTERVENTIONS

Equipment/Supplies

- Electric or safety razor
- Mirror
- Shaving cream or soap
- Basin of warm water
- Bath, hand towel, washcloth
- Shaving lotion
- Disposable gloves

Resident

- Explain purpose of procedure and expected results
- Place a hand towel over the chest to protect clothing
- Place in semi- or high-Fowler's position in bed or sitting in chair

PROCEDURE

1. Perform handwashing.
2. Become familiar with type of shaving equipment and pattern of care, possible contraindication for use of electric razor (oxygen use) or safety razor (bleeding disorder).
3. Put on disposable gloves.
4. Wash face and pat dry.
5. To shave with a safety razor:
   a. Moisten a small towel with warm water and place on the part of the face to be shaved for 1-2 minutes to soften the whiskers.
   b. Apply shaving cream or soapy lather to the face for a smooth removal of the hair without pulling.
   c. Begin shaving the face at the sideburns in the direction of hair growth while holding the razor at a 10 degree angle with the dominant hand and pulling the skin taut with the nondominant hand.

    d. Shave with short and firm strokes turning the head as needed to access hard to reach areas.

    e. Continue shaving down the sides of the face, across the chin, around the mouth, and up the neck.

    f. Rinse the razor in the basin of water periodically and add more shaving cream or lather when needed.

    g. Remove excess shaving cream or lather with a washcloth, change the water, wipe the face, pat dry, and apply after-shave lotion.

    h. Wash razor and store with other articles for further use, discard gloves and place soiled linen in the hamper.

6. To shave with an electric razor:

    a. Inspect the razor and remove any hair left from previous use.

    b. Plug in and set or adjust the shaver head to the desired height.

    c. Apply a pre-shave lotion to clean the skin and have the hair stand erect for easier removal.

    d. Shave in a circular motion applying pressure against the skin and against the hair growth with the shaver in the dominant hand while holding the skin taut with the nondominant hand if using a shaver with rotary blades; in a back and forth motion if using a shaver with straight blades.

    e. Change to shaving in the direction of hair growth on the neck to prevent irritation of these more sensitive areas.

    f. Apply after-shave lotion according to resident preference.

    g. Clean the head of the shaver, store with other articles for future use.

7. Apply an antiseptic to any cuts or nicks in the skin.

❧ PROBLEM-SOLVING ACTIONS

1. Assess electric razor cord for fraying or other safety violations.

2. Avoid shaving if a wound or skin eruption is present on the face.

3. A safety razor should not be used if the resident has a bleeding disorder or is receiving anticoagulant therapy.

4. An electric razor should not be used if the resident is receiving oxygen unless special precautions are taken (grounding, double-insulation on wires).

5. Encourage independence in the shaving procedure by supplying aids such as an extended handle, a larger easier to grasp and hold handle, suction cups to hold tubes or other containers in place while removing the cream or lotion.

6. Provide an over-the-bed table or chair at the sink to promote independence and allow all the time needed for resident to perform the procedure.

❧ EVALUATION

Cleanliness and comfort promoted; skin integrity demonstrated and maintained

VAGINAL IRRIGATION

V*aginal irrigation, also known as vaginal douche, is the introduction of a solution into the vaginal cavity to promote comfort by cleansing and removing excessive discharge and odors, and to provide antiseptics to the area in the treatment or prevention of infection. The normal pH of the vagina is acidic (3.5-4.2) and becomes more alkaline (5.7) at menopause as estrogen levels and mucous production decrease and the tract becomes atrophic with aging. These changes in combination with a thinning of the tissues of the vagina and external genitalia predispose the area to infection. Frequency of the procedure depends on assessment and reason for the procedure. Clean technique is utilized for vaginal irrigation unless lesions or open wounds are present.*

❧ ASSESSMENT

Discharge for amount, color, odor, and consistency, genitalia for redness, pain, itching, irritation, antiseptics to be added to the solution

❧ NURSING DIAGNOSES

High Risk for Impaired Tissue Integrity; Body Image Disturbance; High Risk for Infection

❧ GOAL

Maintain comfort, genitalia and vaginal integrity and cleanliness

❧ INTERVENTIONS

Equipment/Supplies

- Plastic container or bag (disposable or reusable) with tubing and clamp or a douche kit containing all equipment and supplies
- Perforated plastic or glass douche nozzle

- Disposable gloves
- Water-soluble lubricating jelly
- Cotton balls

- Antiseptic solution for cleansing

- Irrigating solution in correct amount and temperature
- IV pole
- Bedpan and tissue
- Waterproof bed protector

Resident

- Explain purpose of procedure and expected results
- Position in dorsal recumbent and drape with bath blanket for privacy

❧ PROCEDURE

1. Perform handwashing.

2. Become familiar with the time and frequency to perform the procedure, the reason for and type of solution and expected results from the procedure.

3. Prepare the solution and equipment, usually about 1000 ml at 96-98° F temperature, hang container on the IV pole 12-24 inches above the hips, and remove the air from the tubing and clamp.

4. Put on disposable gloves and place the protective pad under the hips and the resident comfortably on a bedpan; allow to void into the bedpan before starting the procedure.

5. Cleanse the vulva with cotton balls and antiseptic solution, to remove any secretions and microorganisms that can be introduced into the vagina, with one stroke downward on the center and each side.

6. Hold nozzle in the dominant hand and examine for defects and apply lubricant to the nozzle.

7. Open the clamp and allow a small amount of the solution to flow over the vulva from the top to the bottom with the solution running into the bedpan.

8. Insert the nozzle into the vagina backward and following the anatomic shape of the vagina.

9. Allow the solution to flow as the nozzle is rotated and moved outward and inward in the vagina to reach all areas.

10. Clamp the tubing and remove the nozzle after all solution is used and wipe the genitalia with tissue.

11. Remove the bedpan, dry the perineum and buttocks as needed wiping from front to back.

12. Assist to a position of comfort.

13. Remove gloves and discard with used articles and clean and store reusable supplies according to Universal Precautions.

❧ PROBLEM-SOLVING ACTIONS

1. Forceful insertion of the nozzle can damage the vaginal tissues.

2. Solutions that irritate the vaginal tissues or a high flow pressure can predispose for infection of the uterine cavity.

3. Raising the resident to a high-Fowler's position can help to expel any solution into the bedpan after all the solution has been administered.

4. Readjust the solution temperature if it feels too warm when a small amount is allowed to flow over the vulva before the nozzle is inserted.

5. If partial or all of the procedure can be performed by the resident, offer assistance in preparation and implementation as needed.

❧ EVALUATION

Color and debris in return solution indicating elimination of vaginal abnormalities and odors; comfort and cleanliness status attained

UNIT V

MEDICATION ADMINISTRATION

- Medications, Ear Drops
- Medications, Eye Drops/Ointment
- Medications, Inhalation (Hand Held Metered Dose)
- Medications, Inhalation (Small Volume Nebulizer)
- Medications, Intradermal Injection
- Medications, Intramuscular Injection
- Medications, Mouth/Throat
- Medications, Nasal Drops/Spray

- Medications, Nasogastric/ Gastrostomy Tube
- Medications, Oral Tablet/Liquid
- Medications, Rectal Suppository
- Medications, Skin
- Medications, Subcutaneous Injection
- Medications, Sublingual/Buccal
- Medications, Transdermal
- Medications, Vaginal Suppository/ Cream

MEDICATIONS, EAR DROPS

Ear drops are medications that are instilled into the auditory canal to provide relief of pain, soften cerumen for easier removal, or treat infection or other disorders (local effect). One or both ears may be treated with drops, as well as ointment or a solution of 70% alcohol applied to the pinna to relieve itching. Clean technique is utilized unless the tympanic membrane has been damaged or ruptured or if skin breaks are evident in or around the pinna or canal.

ASSESSMENT

Cerumen in the ear(s); pain in ear with or without drainage; redness, swelling, and discharge in the auditory canal; ruptured or intact tympanic membrane; history of ear infections or other ear disorders

NURSING DIAGNOSES

Pain, High Risk for Infection, Sensory/Perceptual Alterations (Auditory)

GOALS

Relief of discomfort; improvement in ear obstruction or condition; safe and correct instillation/application of drops or ointment

INTERVENTIONS

Equipment/Supplies

- Otic medication in properly-labeled tube or bottle with dropper
- Cotton-tipped applicators or cotton balls
- Tissues, cloth for wiping

Resident

- Explain purpose of procedure and expected results
- Place in sidelying position with ear to be treated in uppermost position

PROCEDURE

1. Perform medication check with medication sheet, physician written order (before preparation, before taking to resident, before administration to resident).
2. Become familiar with drug action, dose, route, side effects, interactions and possible allergic reactions, expected response using a drug reference.
3. Perform handwashing.
4. Take medication and supplies to the bedside.
5. Identify the resident by wristband.
6. Wipe pinna with damp washcloth and external auditory canal orifice with applicator and warm water to remove dried secretions.
7. Hold medication bottle in hand for 2 minutes to warm solution for comfort and to prevent vertigo.
8. Withdraw the medication from the bottle and place into the dropper with the dominant hand.
9. Hold upper part of pinna and pull upward and backward with non-dominant hand to straighten auditory canal.

10. Instill ordered number of drops and gently press on tragus to facilitate passage of the drops into the external auditory canal.

11. Release the pinna, wipe away excess medication and allow the resident to remain in the same position for 3 to 5 minutes.

12. Insert a small cotton plug into the orifice of the canal to retain medication in the ear for 15 to 30 minutes if needed.

13. Change position to other side and repeat procedure to other ear if ordered.

14. If external administration of topical solution is to be done, use cotton applicators or cotton balls with medication and wipe pinna, usually to relieve itching.

15. Remove medication and wipe pinna, to relieve itching.

16. Wash hands.

ᴥ PROBLEM-SOLVING ACTIONS

1. Carefully read otic or optic medications to ensure correct drug use.

2. Place non-dominant hand on head when using the otoscope for examination or when administering the drops into the ear to stabilize the head and prevent injury or contamination of the dropper if the resident should move.

3. Use sterile solutions and aseptic technique to prevent any possible entry of organisms into the middle or inner ear.

4. Gentle handling of the pinna and tragus will prevent additional pain associated with ear infections.

5. Avoid allowing the cotton plug to remain in place longer than 30 minutes as this may affect hearing and predispose to the entry of organism into the canal or inserting cotton-tipped applicator into the ear.

6. Administer other medications, such as antibiotics and analgesics, if ordered.

7. Prepare for ear irrigation for cerumen removal by physician, if appropriate.

ᴥ EVALUATION

Reported feeling of medication in ear and relief of pain, improved hearing after removal of cerumen

MEDICATIONS, EYE DROPS/OINTMENT

Eye drops and ointments are medications that are instilled or applied into the eye(s) to provide treatment for infection, dry eye condition, post-operative cataract care, to dilate the pupils for eye examination, to constrict the pupil for glaucoma, to anesthetize the cornea for tonometry examination, or to reduce irritation caused by allergies or other irritants (local effect). One or both eyes may be treated with drops/ointment. The medication is usually prepared in a dilute solution (less than 1% in strength) and a base that does not irritate sensitive eyes. Sterile technique is utilized for all eye medication administration.

ASSESSMENT

Pain, itching, burning, or blurring of vision in eye(s); redness, discharge, or tearing of eye(s); eyelid swelling; squinting, blinking or rubbing eye(s)

NURSING DIAGNOSES

Pain; High Risk for Infection; Sensory/Perceptual Alterations (Visual)

GOAL

Relief of discomfort; improvement in or optimal vision; absence of infection; safe and correct instillation/application of drops or ointment

INTERVENTIONS

Equipment/Supplies

- Optic medication in properly labeled tube, squeeze bottle, or bottle with dropper
- Sterile gauze squares or cotton balls
- Tissues
- Eye pad dressing, packaged and sterile if needed with paper tape
- Disposable gloves

Resident

- Explain purpose of procedure and expected results
- Place in supine position with the head resting on a small pillow and eye to be treated lower than second eye, or in sitting position if preferred with head hyper-extended

PROCEDURE

1. Perform medication check with medication sheet, physician written order (before preparation, before taking to resident, before administration to resident).
2. Become familiar with the drug action, dose, route, form, side effects, interactions, expected results using a drug reference.
3. Carefully recheck which eye is to be treated.
4. Perform handwashing.
5. Take medication and supplies to the bedside or location of resident providing that privacy is maintained.
6. Identify the resident by wrist band.

7. Cleanse eyelid and around eye with gauze square or cotton ball and sterile saline wiping from the inner to outer canthus; use one square or ball for each wipe.

8. Repeat handwashing; use gloves if contact with secretions is likely.

9. Hold medication bottle or tube in hand for 2 minutes to warm before application.

10. Withdraw the medication from the bottle and place into the dropper or remove the cap on the squeeze bottle or tube with the dominant hand; discard first drop of ointment.

11. Gently place the non-dominant hand with a gauze square or cotton ball on the cheekbone under the eye and pull the skin and lower lid downward exposing the lower conjunctiva.

12. Ask the resident to look upward.

13. While holding the bottle or tube in a vertical position and slightly to the side of the eye and about one-half inches above the eye, instill the ordered number of drops into the conjunctival sac, or a ribbon of ointment along the lower conjunctiva from the inner to outer canthus.

14. Ask the resident to close the eye for 1 to 2 minutes.

15. Wipe excess medication from around the eye with tissue.

16. Apply eye pad dressing if ordered, usually reserved for post-operative care.

17. Reposition and repeat procedure for second eye if appropriate; repeat handwashing first if secretions present.

18. Remove medications for future use, discard used articles.

19. Wash hands.

❧ PROBLEM-SOLVING ACTIONS

1. Carefully read otic or optic medications and check medication to read "ophthalmic" to ensure correct drug use; recheck for correct eye: OD=right eye, OS=left eye, OU=both eyes.

2. Place non-dominant hand on forehead when administering the drops or ointment to stabilize head and prevent injury or contamination of the dropper or tip of squeeze bottle or tube in the event the resident moves during the treatment.

3. Explain to the resident that vision may be blurred for a short time following the administration of ointment but that this is temporary.

4. Ask the resident to avoid squeezing the eye or closing the eye tightly after the medication has been administered as this may expel the medication.

5. If both eyes are to be treated, wash hands between care of each eye, use separate tube or bottle of medication and separate supplies for each eye to prevent the transmission of organisms from one eye to the other; avoid using same container of eye medication for more than one person.

6. Some gentle pressure may be applied over the inner canthus following administration of the medication to increase contact time with the eye tissue for an increased effectiveness of the drug.

7. Discard solution remaining in the dropper before putting it back into the bottle of medication.

8. Provide effective lighting without glare for vision, provide optimal humidity and avoid anything in the environment that dries the eyes, offer vision optical aids such as magnifying devices, glasses, contact lenses, closed circuit TV, special lamps, large print books, newspapers, telephone dials for those with impaired vision.

❧ EVALUATION

Reported relief of eye pain and irritation, vision maintained at optimal level

MEDICATIONS, INHALATION
(HAND HELD METERED DOSE)

Inhalation of medications (INH) into the respiratory tract by hand-held metered dose is usually performed to provide rapid relief from airway congestion, bronchospasms, and to prevent airway inflammation. Decongestants, bronchodilators, and steroids may be given to treat allergic reactions and chronic pulmonary conditions (local effect). An apparatus delivers a measured dose that is inhaled through the nose or mouth by manual compression of a cartridge that causes the medication to enter the airways as air is inhaled. The medication may be contained in a cartridge with series of doses or in a single-dose capsule of a powdered form of the medication administered by a turbo-inhaler. The delivery device may be washed and reused and cartridges replaced when empty per order. Clean technique is utilized for inhalation medication administration.

❧ ASSESSMENT

Breathing difficulty with respiratory rate, depth, and ease, pulse rate, history of allergic or pulmonary conditions or diseases

❧ NURSING DIAGNOSES

Ineffective Breathing Pattern; High Risk for Infection

❧ GOALS

Relief and control of difficulty in breathing; safe and correct administration of medication via the inhalation route

❧ INTERVENTIONS

Equipment/Supplies

- Medication in properly-labeled, metered dose cartridge or unit dose package with dispenser
- Mouthwash, glass of water

- Tissues, basin

Resident

- Explain purpose of procedure and expected results
- Place in upright sitting position

❧ PROCEDURE

1. Perform medication check with medication sheet, physician written order (before preparation, before taking to resident, before administration to resident).
2. Become familiar with the drug action, dose, route, form, side effects, interactions, expected results using a drug reference.
3. Perform handwashing.
4. Place the cartridge into the dispenser and shake well to distribute the propellent.

5. Remove cap from the mouthpiece and ask resident to open mouth; place it in the mouth that is slightly opened or with lips around the mouthpiece.

6. Ask resident to exhale, then inhale slowly while compressing the cartridge firmly in the holder to release a dose of the medication; hold breath for 5 seconds, or as long as able.

7. Remove mouthpiece and breath normally, repeat procedure for a second dose or as ordered.

8. If a nasal inhaler is used, perform same procedure by placing the tip into a naris while holding the other naris closed with a finger and repeat on the opposite side.

9. For unit dose powdered medication using a turbo-inhaler device (which delivers the medication by the force of inhaled air), place the capsule of the medication in the inhaler and follow the steps taken for metered dose cartridge and repeat inhalations until all of the medication has been inhaled.

10. Perform mouth care or rinse, offer tissues to wipe mouth.

11. Note changes in pulse (tachycardia) following each inhalation dose of medication.

12. Remove cartridge if used; rinse or wash inhaler device as needed and allow to air dry.

13. Remove medication or store at resident's bedside for future use.

14. Wash hands.

✍ PROBLEM-SOLVING ACTIONS

1. When the medication in the cartridge is almost gone, amount and effect of drug may decrease.

2. Various assistive devices are available to promote medication inhalation for those who have difficulty using the hand-held apparatus effectively.

3. Check cartridge for punctures before using.

4. Inform resident of danger in overuse of inhalants which can cause severe side effects or decrease the effectiveness of the medication.

5. Caution the resident to inhale the medication and to avoid exhaling into the device.

6. Supervise and evaluate self-administration of hand-held metered dose inhalants with medication kept at bedside for immediate access and use by resident.

7. Provide mouthwash, rinse following use of inhalants, if desired, or as definitely required if steroids are being administered.

8. Allow resident to carry inhaler in a pocket for quick relief or prevention of breathing difficulty.

✍ EVALUATION

Respiratory rate, depth, and ease within baseline parameters, reduced respiratory congestion and allergic reactions

MEDICATIONS, INHALATION
(SMALL VOLUME NEBULIZER)

Inhalation of medications into the respiratory tract by small volume nebulizer (SVN) is usually performed to provide relief from airway congestion, bronchospasms, and to liquify and mobilize secretions for easier removal. Decongestants, bronchodilators, and mucolytics may be given to treat allergic and chronic pulmonary conditions and diseases (local effect). A machine provides a stream of air that produces a suspension of fine particles that is inhaled through the mouth into the trachea, bronchi, and alveolar spaces. The medication is placed in a container attached to the machine by tubing and held in a hand during administration. The stream of air is forced into the container and converts the liquid medication into aerosol that escapes through an attached mouthpiece when inhalation takes place. The containers may be washed, disinfected and reused unless defective from prolonged use. Clean technique is utilized for inhalation medication administration although the solution of medication, whether unit dose or stock bottle, is sterile.

❧ ASSESSMENT

Breathing difficulty with respiratory rate and depth; increased pulse rate, history of allergies or pulmonary conditions, inability to cough up mucous

❧ NURSING DIAGNOSES

Ineffective Breathing Pattern; Ineffective Airway Clearance; High Risk for Infection

❧ GOALS

Relief and control of breathing difficulty; airway patency; safe and correct administration of medication via the inhalation route

❧ INTERVENTIONS

Equipment\Supplies

- Medication in properly labeled unit dose or bottle
- Small volume nebulizer
- Tubing and medication cup complete with parts
- Medicine cup for measuring medication, if needed
- Tissues, mouthwash, basin
- Stethoscope

Resident

- Explain purpose of procedure and expected results
- Place in upright sitting position or as near sitting as comfortable

❧ PROCEDURE

1. Perform medication check with medication sheet, physician written order (before preparation, before taking to resident, before administration to resident).
2. Become familiar with the drug action, dose, route, form, side effects, interactions, expected results using a drug reference.

3. Perform handwashing.

4. Plug machine into an electric outlet; attach tubing to the proper outlet on the machine.

5. Pour correct amount of medication and sterile normal saline into medicine cup for measurement or uncap unit dose bottle.

6. Remove cover from cup attached to other end of the tubing and pour medication into it.

7. Recap the cup and attach mouthpiece.

8. Turn on the machine and place the mouthpiece into resident's mouth and request to close the lips around it.

9. Request resident to breathe normally with a deep breath taken every fourth breath, continue for 10 to 15 minutes.

10. Remove mouthpiece when all medication has been inhaled, check pulse and breath sounds with stethoscope.

11. Provide mouthwash or drink of water if desired.

12. Turn machine off and disconnect cup from tubing; wash, rinse cup and parts, and allow to air dry.

13. Submerge cup and all parts in a disinfectant solution weekly or according to agency policies depending on frequency of use, rinse well and allow to air dry.

14. Store medication and supplies for future use or allow machine to remain at bedside if appropriate.

15. Wash hands.

❧ PROBLEM SOLVING ACTIONS

1. Supervise and evaluate self-administration of inhalation of medications by SVN and caution against administration of more medication than physician ordered or more frequently than ordered.

2. Maintain machine in the off position and unplug from outlet when not in use; follow manufacturer's instructions for care of machine.

3. A variety of different medicine cups used in SVN treatments are available; follow instructions on the package to assemble for use.

❧ EVALUATION

Respiratory rate, depth, and ease within baseline parameters, ability to cough up mucous and clear airway, absence of respiratory infection

MEDICATIONS, INTRADERMAL INJECTION

Intradermal medications are administered by injection into the skin between the epidermis and dermis layers. The route is used to administer medication to test for allergies or to determine susceptibility, resistance or immune competence to specific diseases. The most common site for this type of injection is the inner aspects of the forearm about 3 inches below the antecubital space. Another site such as the back of the thigh can also be used if the arms are not available or cannot be used because of skin eruptions. Most medications administered via this route are available in a vial and administered by a tuberculin syringe because very small amounts are injected, usually no more than 0.1 ml. Sterile technique is utilized for all procedures associated with medication administration by the intradermal route.

❧ ASSESSMENT

Skin at the selected site for breaks, rash or other eruptions, reason for injection and expected possible results, history of allergies and infectious diseases

❧ NURSING DIAGNOSES

High Risk for Infection; Anxiety; Pain

❧ GOALS

Safe and correct administration of test substance via the intradermal route

❧ INTERVENTIONS

Equipment/Supplies

- Medication in a vial properly labeled
- Sterile tuberculin syringe with attached needle
- Antiseptic and acetone swabs
- Biohazard puncture-resistant container for disposal

Resident

- Explain purpose of procedure and expected results
- Place in a comfortable position with arm supported and site exposed

❧ PROCEDURE

1. Perform medication check with medication sheet, physician written order (before preparation, before taking to resident, before administration to resident).

2. Become familiar with purpose of the test, action, side effects, expected response using a drug reference.

3. Perform handwashing.

4. Remove syringe with attached needle from the package or, if packaged separately, attach the needle with the cover in place and maintaining sterile technique.

5. Remove the metal cap and/or cover from the vial and cleanse the top with an antiseptic swab.

6. Remove the needle cover and place in a clean area, withdraw the volume of air that is the same as the volume of medication to be withdrawn from the vial, only touch the barrel tip of the plunger on the syringe.

7. Puncture the vial diaphragm with the needle and expel the air into the vial above the level of the medication and, while holding the vial upright and the needle tip covered by the solution with the nondominant hand, withdraw the entire or measured amount of medication into the syringe with the dominant hand.

8. Withdraw the needle from the vial and expel air leaving 0.1 less of air to clear the needle during injection; place the prepared syringe in a clean area and prevent contamination of the needle.

9. Take the prepared medication to the resident, identify by wristband.

10. Cleanse the site(s) with acetone swab to remove oil and other substances from the skin.

11. Support the forearm with the nondominant hand and stretch the skin taut.

12. Hold the syringe in the dominant hand with the needle as parallel as possible to the skin (15 degree angle) with the bevel side upward.

13. Insert the needle under the skin surface until the bevel is within the skin and carefully palpate to identify the ridge of the needle to ensure that the injection is not too deep.

14. Slowly inject the medication and note the formation of a bleb on the skin.

15. Withdraw the needle after the medication has been injected and wipe the site with an antiseptic swab; do not massage the area.

16. Circle the area(s) of infection on the skin or prepare a chart of the injection(s) with the identifying information.

17. Inspect the site at the appropriate time, usually 24-72 hours depending on the type of test, to determine a positive or negative response.

18. If the response is positive, measure the diameter, erythema and induration of the response.

19. Discard the used articles in a biohazard container with needle uncovered and attached to the syringe.

20. Wash hands.

❧ PROBLEM-SOLVING ACTIONS

1. Gloves should be worn according to Universal Precautions.

2. Good lighting assists in performing the procedure and visualization of the needle ridge under the skin.

3. If the needle ridge is not palpable or visualized or is movable under the skin, withdraw slightly and reinsert it more superficially.

4. If a bleb does not form when the medication is injected, remove the needle from the injection site as it has been inserted too deeply, prepare another syringe and repeat the procedure.

❧ EVALUATION

Successful administration of medication(s) via the intradermal injection route without incident

MEDICATIONS, INTRAMUSCULAR INJECTION

Intramuscular medications (IM) are administered by injection into a muscle mass which is selected based on the amount of drug to be injected and the desired rate of absorption. The age, size of muscle mass, and physical condition of the resident are also considerations for the determination of injection sites. The most common sites used are the upper arm in the deltoid muscle and dorsal gluteal area in the gluteus maximus muscle. Medication that is injected into a muscle is absorbed into the circulation (systemic effect), metabolized by the liver, and excreted by the kidneys and is given by this route when residents are unable to take it orally or the medication cannot produce the desired effect when given orally. Because muscle is a highly-vascular tissue, medications injected intramuscularly produce a more rapid action than other injections into tissues or those administered via the subcutaneous or oral routes. The maximum volume of solution injected into the muscle tissue is usually 2.5 ml. Medications for injection are available in sterile, one-dose ampules, pre-filled cartridges, and multiple-dose sterile vials. Sterile technique is utilized for all medication administration by intramuscular injection.

ASSESSMENT

Possible site for muscle mass that is healthy and adequate for proposed depth of injection, site of last injection, drug allergies, compatibility of mixed medications, age and weight, general health and circulation status

NURSING DIAGNOSES

Pain; High Risk for Injury; Impaired Tissue Integrity

GOALS

Safe and correct administration of medication via the intramuscular route

INTERVENTIONS

Equipment/Supplies

- Medication in vial or ampule properly labeled 2 to 3 ml syringe in sterile package
- Needles of appropriate size for depth 1 to 2 ½ inches and appropriate gauge for solution from 20 to 23; packaged sterile separately or attached to the syringe
- Small metal file
- Metal device or holder for pre-filled cartridge unit

- Sponges with antiseptic
- Sterile water or normal saline for injection if needed as diluents
- Bandaid
- Biohazard container for proper disposal

Resident

- Explain purpose of procedure and expected results
- Place in sidelying, sitting or dorsal position depending on site to be used and drape to expose area as needed

❧ PROCEDURE

1. Perform medication check with medication sheet, physician written order (before preparation, before taking to resident, before administration to resident).

2. Become familiar with drug action, dose, route, side effects, interactions, expected response using a drug reference.

3. Determine appropriate syringe and needle for medication to be administered and site to be used.

4. Perform handwashing.

5. Remove syringe from package, attach needle if packaged separately maintaining sterile technique and needle with cover in place.

6. Remove the metal cap or cover on the vial or multi-dose reused vial and cleanse the rubber diaphragm with an antiseptic.

7. Place the prepared medication in a clean place and withdraw the volume of air that is the same as the volume of medication to be withdrawn from the vial while careful not to touch anything but the syringe barrel and tip of the plunger.

8. Puncture vial diaphragm with the needle and expel the air into the vial above the level of the medication; while holding vial upright and needle tip covered by the solution with the non-dominant hand, withdraw the entire or measured amount of medication into the syringe with the dominant hand.

9. Withdraw needle from vial and expel air leaving 0.1 to 0.2 ml to clear needle of the medication during the injection.

10. Replace needle cover and place with the identifying medication sheet or card.

11. If pre-filled cartridge is used, assemble the cartridge in the holder and leave cover on needle.

12. If ampule of medication is used, ensure that solution is not in stem of ampule by shaking or flicking with the finger; cleanse ampule with antiseptic sponge and snap off with fingers if neck is scored; if not scored, use the metal file on the neck of the ampule and snap off.

13. Insert uncovered needle held with dominant hand into the ampule held with the nondominant hand between the index and middle fingers and withdraw the medication without allowing the needle to touch the sides of the neck of the ampule.

14. Hold syringe upright to expel all but 0.1 to 0.2 ml of air, use the empty ampule for identification of medication before administering.

15. If medication needs to be reconstituted, follow directions on the package insert for amounts of diluent to use for desired dosage and prepare for administration as with the vial procedure.

16. Take prepared medication to bedside, identify the resident by wrist-band.

17. Palpate and identify site with hands.

18. Pickup syringe and hold in dominant hand.

19. Cleanse site with antiseptic sponge and spread skin taut with non-dominant hand.

20. Insert the needle at a 90° angle with smooth, firm motion.

21. Hold syringe with nondominant hand and aspirate for possible puncture into a blood vessel by noting blood in the syringe.

22. Inject medication into the muscle slowly, no more than 1 ml/4 seconds.

23. Place antiseptic sponge at side of needle, apply slight pressure and withdraw needle, apply pressure and massage site gently.

24. Apply bandaid if needed or additional pressure if bleeding occurs.

25. Discard syringe with needle attached in biohazard container according to Universal Precautions.

26. Discard other used articles or store for further use if appropriate.

27. Wash hands.

❧ PROBLEM-SOLVING ACTIONS

1. Perform assessment required for specific medications (Z-track, preparations in oil.)

2. Using the smallest gauge and sharpest needle possible and performing the procedure quickly and efficiently will reduce pain and anxiety associated with this procedure; inform resident of those medications that cause burning sensations or pain.

3. Additional pressure is needed at the site if resident is taking anticoagulant therapy.

4. Note drug labeling for the route to be used before administering as complications may occur if improper route is used for a particular drug.

5. Powdered drug preparations are reconstituted with the volume and type of diluent and the strength or concentration of the drug as identified on the label or the insert; the volume of the diluent is usually less than the reconstituted volume because of the displacement from the powdered form of the drug.

6. Gloves should be worn in those cases where Universal Precautions dictate.

7. Promote resident relaxation as the needle enters tissue more easily when muscles are relaxed.

8. Careless handling of a used needle may transmit infectious diseases from the resident to the nurse.

9. If blood is noted in the syringe when withdrawing the plunger after inserting the needle, withdraw the needle, discard the syringe and begin the procedure again.

10. Sign appropriate forms when administering controlled substances.

11. Store parenteral medications in appropriate manner, medication cart, medication room, refrigerator, room temperature.

12. If medications are to be combined in one syringe, check on compatibilities and note any reaction in the mixed solution.

13. Premixed and measured medications in a cartridge should be administered according to the manufacturer's instructions.

❧ EVALUATION

Successful administration of medications via the intramuscular injection route without incident

MEDICATIONS, MOUTH/THROAT

Mouth and throat medications are administered by spray, mouthwash, gargling, swabbing, or lozenges which provide treatment for pain, inflammation, infection, or to reduce sensation (local effect). Medications used include antiseptics, antimicrobials, astringents, and anesthetics. Lozenges or troches are large tablets that dissolve in the mouth to treat throat irritation and pain. Mouth and throat sprays treat irritation and anesthetize the mucosa to reduce discomfort or prepare for treatment. Mouthwashes and gargles provide treatments for infections, inflammation, and pain with the solution expectorated after swishing or holding it in the mouth. Swabbing the mouth or throat may prove an alternate for application of medications if the other methods cannot be utilized or if the resident is unable to perform them. Clean technique is utilized for mouth and throat medication administration.

ASSESSMENT

Mouth or throat irritation or pain, lesions, inflammation or infectious process of the mouth, ability to perform procedure, fit and adequacy of dentures

NURSING DIAGNOSES

Pain; High Risk for Infection; Altered Oral Mucous Membrane

GOALS

Relief of pain or discomfort; improved condition of oral cavity; safe and correct administration of medication via the method utilized

INTERVENTIONS

Equipment/Supplies

- Medication in proper form and labeling in medicine cup or container
- Cotton-tipped applicators, tongue depressor
- Basin, tissues
- Flashlight or penlight
- Disposable gloves

Resident

- Explain purpose of procedure and expected results
- Remove full or partial dentures
- Place in semi-Fowler's or sitting position

PROCEDURE

1. Perform medication check with medication sheet, physician written order (before preparation, before taking to resident, before administration to resident).
2. Become familiar with the drug action, dose, route, form, side effects, interactions, and expected results using the drug reference.
3. Determine which method of administration is to be used.
4. Perform handwashing.

5. If a solution, prepare the medication in the proper container for administration (glass, spray pump, atomizer, medicine cup with calibrated measurement).

6. Take the medication to the resident.

7. Identify resident by wristband.

8. Remove lozenge from wrapper or bottle and request the resident to place tablet in the mouth; advise to swallow the medication after it has mixed with the saliva until it completely dissolves and not to chew or swallow it whole.

9. To administer medication via pump spray or atomizer, request the resident to open the mouth and inspect it by compressing the tongue with a tongue depressor.

10. Hold the nozzle of a spray pump just outside the mouth, or insert the tip of the atomizer inside the mouth, and direct the spray toward the back of the throat.

11. Press the pump nozzle or atomizer bulb firmly with pressure that will propel the medication to the area to be treated, request the resident to refrain from swallowing or drinking water after spraying.

12. To administer medication via gargling, request the resident to take 30 ml or less of the solution into the mouth and tilt the head slightly backwards allowing the liquid to run back into the throat; to create a gargle by exhaling slowly through the mouth, expectorate the solution into a sink or basin, wipe mouth with tissue and repeat as needed.

13. To administer medication via mouthwash, request the resident to take 30 ml or less of the solution into the mouth and swish it throughout the mouth, gums, and teeth, expectorate the solution into the sink or basin, wipe the mouth with tissue and repeat as needed; for some medications the resident may be asked to hold the medication in the mouth as long as possible after swishing action and then swallow it.

14. Remove medication and clean supplies for future use and store; discard used tissues.

15. Wash hands.

❧ PROBLEM-SOLVING ACTIONS

1. Stabilize head with nondominant hand during spraying procedure if needed.

2. Topical anesthetics may interfere with swallowing, so food and fluid may be withheld for 1 hour following administration.

3. Solutions for mouthwash and gargle should be warmed to room temperature.

4. A drink of water should be offered before a spraying procedure as this may be contraindicated after the treatment.

5. If aspiration of medication is a possibility, remain with resident until sensation returns.

6. Medications that are swallowed may result in a systemic effect and this should be monitored for untoward responses or overdosage.

7. If dentures are worn, remove until condition of mouth improves except for meals.

❧ EVALUATIONS

Reported relief of pain or discomfort, improved condition of oral and throat mucosa

MEDICATIONS, NASAL DROPS/SPRAY

Nasal drops and sprays are medications that are instilled or sprayed into the nose to provide treatment for blocked or congested nasal or sinus passages, and to reduce inflammation of the nasal mucosa (local effect). Nasal sprays are also used for conditions in which absorption of the drug provides a desired effect when the drug would be digested if taken orally as in vasopressin prescribed for the treatment of diabetes insipidus (systemic effect). The medication is usually prepared in an isotonic aqueous solution that does not irritate the sensitive mucosa of the nasal cavity. Clean technique is utilized for nasal medication administration.

ASSESSMENT

Nasal congestion, difficulty breathing through the nose, redness of the nasal mucosa, thick, viscous nasal discharge, dry nasal passages, history of nasal allergies and chronic use of nasal medications

NURSING DIAGNOSES

High Risk for Infection; Sensory/Perceptual Alterations (Olfactory); Ineffective Breathing Pattern

GOALS

Relief of nasal stuffiness and congestion; absence of infection; improved nasal breathing; safe and correct instillation/application of drops or spray

INTERVENTIONS

Equipment/Supplies

- Nasal medication in properly labeled squeeze bottle or bottle with dropper
- Tissues, cotton-tipped applicators

- Nasal speculum if appropriate
- Disposable gloves

Resident

- Explain purpose of procedure and expected results
- Place in supine or sitting position with head hyperextended and small pillow under the shoulders; or over the edge of the bed for medication to reach the sinuses

PROCEDURE

1. Perform medication check with medication sheet, physician written order (before preparation, before taking to resident, before administration to resident).
2. Become familiar with the drug action, dose, route, form, side effects, interactions, and expected results using a drug reference.
3. Determine if drops or spray is to be administered.
4. Perform handwashing.
5. Take medication and supplies to the resident.
6. Identify the resident by wristband.
7. Put on gloves, request the resident to blow nose and cleanse secretions away from the nasal area with a tissue or cotton-tipped applicator.

8. Withdraw the medication into the dropper with the dominant hand or uncap the spray or squeeze bottle if this is the type of dispenser used.

9. Gently raise the tip of the nose with the thumb of nondominant hand and ask the resident to breathe through the mouth.

10. Carefully insert the dropper tip just inside the nasal passage without touching the sides and holding it horizontally to the nose, administer 3 to 4 drops or the amount ordered into the upper and center of both nares.

11. Request the resident to remain in the position for 2 minutes to allow the medication to act on the anterior mucosa and allow subsequent drops to reach posterior mucosa.

12. Repeat instillation of 3 to 4 drops into both nares.

13. Perform same procedure with hyperextension of the neck over the edge of the bed for instillation of medication into the sinuses; support of the head with the nondominant hand.

14. For nasal spray administration, insert the tip of the bottle into each nostril about one-half inch and squeeze the bottle with moderate force once or twice according to prescribed amount; request the resident to remain in the position for 4 to 5 minutes and refrain from blowing the nose; repeat procedure once as needed.

15. Wipe excess medication from the nasal area or give resident a tissue to wipe nose.

16. Remove medications for future use, discard used tissues.

17. Wash hands.

❧ PROBLEM-SOLVING ACTIONS

1. Position correctly with head and neck supported in order for medication to reach desired area to be treated and prevent medication from running down the throat.

2. Avoid use of nasal medications that have an oily base as inhalation of lipids may cause pneumonia or other respiratory infections.

3. Some elderly may not be able to maintain the necessary position for a second administration of the nose drops and may better tolerate a spray, which should be administered in a sitting position with the head slightly tilted backward.

4. For a resident who is unable to remain still or is uncooperative; attach a small rubber tube to the end of the dropper to prevent injury to the mucosa.

5. It is recommended that enough medication be withdrawn for both nares rather than reintroduce the dropper into the bottle during the procedure.

6. Provide humification of room air by cold mist to promote nasal drainage and prevent nasal mucosa dryness and irritation (see Breathing Therapy Devices).

7. If using an aerosol spray, avoid puncture or damage to the cartridge and store at room temperature.

❧ EVALUATION

Reported relief of nasal congestion, irritation

MEDICATIONS, NASOGASTRIC/GASTROSTOMY TUBE

Nasogastric (NG) or gastrostomy medications are administered through a tube inserted manually or surgically for the purpose of feeding those who are unable to take nourishment by mouth. The same guidelines are applied to medications given via a tube as those given orally. They can be administered by gravity or push method regardless of whether the feedings are intermittent or continuous. Clean technique is utilized for nasogastric or gastrostomy medication administration.

ASSESSMENT

Condition of skin around stoma (gastrostomy) and nasal mucous membrane (nasogastric), toleration of feedings, placement of tube in stomach

NURSING DIAGNOSES

High Risk for Impaired Skin or Mucous Membrane Integrity; High Risk for Aspiration; Body Image Disturbance

GOALS

Retention and tolerance of medication; absence of skin or mucous membrane breakdown; safe and correct instillation of medication via tube

INTERVENTIONS

Equipment/Supplies

- Medication in proper form and labeling in medicine cup or container
- Bulb or catheter syringe or funnel (50 ml)
- Calibrated container with 60 ml water
- Pill crusher or mortar and pestle
- Clamp or cap for tubing
- Stethoscope
- Towel

Resident

- Explain purpose of procedure and expected results
- Place in semi to high Fowler's position as tolerated

PROCEDURE

1. Perform medication check with medication sheet, physician written order (before preparation, before taking to resident, before administration to resident).
2. Become familiar with the drug action, dose, route, form, side effects, interactions, expected results using the drug reference.
3. Perform handwashing.
4. Determine drug form and empty capsule into medicine cup, crush tablet and place in a medicine cup and dissolve in a small amount of water; avoid crushing sustained release tablets or attempting to empty gelcaps.
5. Determine if medication should be administered with or without food and schedule to give between or during feedings.

6. Take the medication to the bedside.

7. Identify resident by wristband.

8. Place small towel over chest to protect clothing.

9. Discontinue continuous feeding if appropriate, place end of tube on towel and clamp.

10. Check placement of tube in stomach by insertion of air into tube and listening to the epigastric area with a stethoscope for a bubbling sound and aspirate contents of stomach with a catheter syringe.

11. Attach the barrel of the syringe to the tube, raise 6 inches above gastrostomy site or at same height as nose for nasogastric site and pour 60 ml water into the syringe; instill and add the liquid or diluted medication to the syringe before all of the water has been instilled; allow to flow into the tube by gravity or administer by push method; amount of fluid used should be ordered.

12. Pour an additional 30 to 60 ml of water into the tube and instill to clear the tube of the medication and to administer the total dosage into the stomach; amount of fluid should be ordered.

13. Remove the syringe and clamp the tubing if appropriate or reattach to continuous feeding administration set if appropriate and unclamp the tubing.

14. Allow the resident to remain in the same position for 30 minutes.

15. Remove supplies and cleanse for future use.

16. Wash hands.

❧ PROBLEM-SOLVING TECHNIQUES

1. Request the physician to write order for liquid form of medication, if available.

2. Administer the medication at a time other than at feeding time if feedings are not well tolerated or absorbed or if a possible formula medication interaction exists (curdling).

3. Use water at room temperature when used in medication administration via tube.

4. Dilute medications that are irritating to the stomach with an increased amount of fluid as with potassium replacement; amount of diluent must be ordered by the physician.

5. Add amount of fluid taken with medications to I&O if this is monitored.

6. If several medications are to be administered, prepare each and mix those that are compatible with water or prepare separately with water and give together or consecutively; amount of fluid should be limited to order regardless of number of medications administered.

7. Provide skin and mucous membrane protection (topical preparation) to prevent irritation from pressure or secretions.

❧ EVALUATION

Tube properly placed in stomach and medication administered correctly, skin and mucous membrane intact and free of irritation or excoriation, no food/medication interaction

MEDICATIONS, ORAL TABLET/LIQUID

O ral (PO) medications are administered in tablet (time-release, enteric coated), capsule, and liquid forms that are available in packaged or unit dose containers or stock supply. They are swallowed and absorbed into the circulation from the gastrointestinal tract to treat or prevent conditions known to have a positive effect from the specific drug therapy (systemic effect). The oral route is the most common and preferred route for medication administration. Clean technique is utilized for oral medication administration.

❧ ASSESSMENT

Dysphagia, drug allergies, condition/illness being treated, history of gastrointestinal conditions affecting ingestion, digestion or absorption, compatibility of medications being administered

❧ NURSING DIAGNOSES

Impaired Swallowing; High Risk for Injury

❧ GOALS

Safe and correct administration of medication via the oral route

❧ INTERVENTIONS

Equipment/Supplies

- Medication in proper form and labeling in unit dose or stock container
- Calibrated medicine cup, souffle cup
- Pill crusher, mortar and pestle
- Syringe with tubing attached to tip
- Water or food to mix with medication
- Glass of water with straw

Resident

- Explain procedure and expected results
- Place in semi Fowler's or sitting position as comfortable

❧ PROCEDURE

1. Perform medication check with medication sheet, physician written order.
   - For unit dose: When removing package from resident supply, before placing package in medicine cup, before opening package at bedside and giving to resident
   - For stock supply: When removing from resident's storage drawer or stock supply of medication, after pouring, measuring liquid or placing tablets in medicine cup, before returning stock supply to storage drawer or cabinet and taking to bedside with medication card or order form

2. Become familiar with drug action, dose, route, side effects, interactions, expected response using a drug reference.

3. Determine need for crushing tablet, emptying of capsule and mixing with liquid or soft food according to physician order and prepare appropriately, do not break enteric-coated or crush time-release tablets or capsules.

4. Perform handwashing.

5. Take prepared medication to bedside and provide a glass of water with or without straw.

6. Identify the resident by wristband.

7. Open package and place medicine cup or tablet in resident's hand or medicine cup of liquid medication in resident's hand.

8. Allow to take some water if mouth is dry and inform resident to take tablets by placing them on the back of the tongue with the head slightly flexed and swallow with water, place capsule on front of tongue and swallow while drinking water.

9. If unable to take medications without assistance, place tablet in mouth or liquid to lips and allow to swallow or use a syringe to administer; request order for medication in liquid form if unable to swallow tablet or capsule.

10. Wait for resident to swallow all medications.

11. Discard used articles.

12. Wash hands.

PROBLEM-SOLVING ACTIONS

1. Perform assessment required for specific medication, usually vital signs.

2. Sign appropriate forms when administering controlled substances.

3. Store medications in appropriate manner, resident's drawer, medication cart, medication room, refrigerator, or at room temperature.

4. Unused or excess medications are never turned to stock or individual supplies.

5. For residents who have trouble swallowing, solid medications may be crushed (if not contraindicated) and added to food. Liquid medications may be administered by syringe with a tubing attached to the tip and inserted between the cheek and teeth and slowly released.

6. Crush tablets with physician order using a pill crushing device, mortar and pestles, or between 2 souffle cups.

7. Offer medications one at a time or all at once, according to resident preference.

8. A full glass of water, unless contraindicated, is recommended for resident when taking oral medications.

9. Note and record fluid intake with medications and I & O is being monitored.

10. Hyperextending the neck causes narrowing of the pharynx and more difficulty in swallowing medications.

11. Only allow crushing or chewing of tablets that would not affect a protective coating or alter release of medication and cause untoward effects or overdose.

12. Unless medications are self-administered, do not leave medications at the bedside or unattended.

13. Discontinue medication and consult physician if side effects occur or order is questioned or secure change of medication order if needed (liquid form, dosage, allergic or other reaction or untoward effect).

EVALUATION

Successful administration of medications via the oral route without incident

MEDICATIONS, RECTAL SUPPOSITORY

A rectal suppository (SUPP) is a medication that is inserted into the rectum to provide stimulation and to promote defecation (local effect) or to treat pain, nausea and vomiting, or to induce relaxation and sedation (systemic effect) when oral administration is not possible or if the drug is rendered ineffective by digestive secretions. The suppository contains the drug prepared with a firm base of glycerin, cocoa butter, lanolin, or gelatin that melts at body temperature.

ASSESSMENT

Hard formed, dry feces; decreased frequency or absence of bowel elimination following administration of a stool softener or bulk forming medications; history of reduced peristalsis, fecal impaction

NURSING DIAGNOSES

Constipation; Constipated, Perceived

GOALS

Bowel elimination without straining; safe and correct insertion of suppository

INTERVENTIONS

Equipment/Supplies

- Suppository in properly labeled, sealed package
- Disposable glove/finger cot
- Water-soluble lubricant

- Bed protector
- Bedpan and tissue if needed
- Light source

Resident

- Explain purpose of procedure and expected results
- Place in sidelying position (left) and drape to expose buttocks

- Provide privacy
- Place light source directed at buttocks

PROCEDURE

1. Perform medication check with medication sheet, physician written order (before preparation, before taking to resident, before administration to resident).
2. Become familiar with drug action, dose, route, side effects, interactions, expected response using a drug reference.
3. Perform handwashing.
4. Take medication and supplies to the bedside.
5. Identify the resident by wristband.
6. Place glove or finger cot on dominant hand or finger.
7. Remove suppository from package and hold in gloved hand.
8. Lubricate tapered tip of suppository if not prelubricated.

9. Separate buttocks with nondominant hand.

10. Gently touch anus with suppository and ask resident to take deep breath.

11. Insert suppository with gloved or cotted finger using gentle pressure in the direction of the umbilicus.

12. Continue insertion of the suppository until it passes the internal anal sphincter (about 1½-2 inches).

13. Remove finger and hold buttocks together for a minute.

14. Cleanse anal area with tissue to remove excess lubricant.

15. Encourage resident to retain suppository for 15 to 20 minutes or until cramping occurs indicating absorption and action of the medication.

16. Remove glove or finger cot and discard with other used, disposable articles in designated container.

17. Place on bedpan in comfortable position or assist to commode/bathroom if given for bowel elimination.

18. Wash hands.

PROBLEM-SOLVING ACTIONS

1. Administer before meals if given for constipation and between meals if given for retention of medication.

2. Place suppository in wrapper under cold running water or in refrigerator if softened.

3. Use additional lubricant if hemorrhoids or other rectal problems are present.

4. Avoid inserting the suppository into fecal mass; insert along side of bowel for desired effect by action on or absorption by mucosa.

5. Hold buttocks together after insertion to prevent accidental expulsion of suppository if the rectal sphincters are weak and function ineffectively to retain it.

6. Provide tissues for cleansing.

7. Provide deodorant to remove room odors if needed.

8. Increase fluid intake, physical activity, and fiber in the diet if appropriate and allowed.

9. Place call light within reach for assistance if needed

EVALUATION

Successful bowel evacuation; relief from discomfort caused by constipation; reduction of temperature, nausea if administered to relieve these

MEDICATIONS, SKIN

Topical (TOP) skin medications are applied externally to provide protection from skin breakdown, lubrication, treat infections of the skin, relieve pruritus and irritation (local effect). They may be applied in the form of powders, lotions, creams, pastes, ointments, or sprays. Types of medications include antiseptics, astringents, antibiotics, and emollients. Clean technique is utilized for topical application unless there are breaks or lesions present which would require sterile technique.

ASSESSMENT

Skin intact or breaks present, redness, dryness, irritation, inflammation, lesions of skin, complaints of itching, burning, history of skin side effects caused by medications

NURSING DIAGNOSES

High Risk for Impaired Skin Integrity; Impaired Skin Integrity; Body Image Disturbance

GOAL

Relief of pruritus or other skin disorder, skin intact and free of changes leading to impaired integrity

INTERVENTIONS

Equipment/Supplies

- Medication in proper form and labeling in proper container
- Sterile and/or nonsterile disposable gloves
- Tongue blades, gauze sponges, applicator swabs
- Sterile dressings, tape
- Bed protector, paper towels
- Warm water, pH neutral cleanser, towel

Resident

- Explain purpose of procedure and expected results
- Remove dressings if present and dispose of appropriately
- Place in position to expose area to be treated, drape if necessary

PROCEDURE

1. Perform medication check with medication sheet, physician written order (before preparation, before taking to resident, before administration to resident).
2. Become familiar with the drug action, amount, route, form, side effects, expected results using the drug reference.
3. Determine which type of preparation to be applied and whether sterile or clean technique is needed.
4. Perform handwashing.
5. Take the medication to the bedside, identify the resident by wristband.
6. Put on sterile or clean disposable gloves.

7. Remove dressing if present and discard properly or cleanse proposed site with warm water and cleanser; pat dry if skin is intact.

8. Remove gloves and wash hands, put on sterile or clean gloves as appropriate.

9. Pour lotion or shake powder in hand and apply to area of skin in the direction of hair growth.

10. Use tongue blade or squeeze tube and place medication on gauze sponge when applying an ointment or paste.

11. Spread evenly over the skin.

12. If spray is used, hold container upright 6 to 12 inches from the area, spray evenly over the surface to be covered.

13. Apply clean, sterile dressing if appropriate and tape.

14. Provide protection to clothing if preparation is needed.

15. Remove medication for future use and dispose of used supplies in designated container.

16. Wash hands.

❧ PROBLEM-SOLVING ACTIONS

1. If a preparation must be removed from its container, use a sterile tongue blade or glove to prevent contamination.

2. If lotions or sprays are used, shake the container before application according to directions.

3. Avoid the application of any skin preparation near the eyes if the face is being treated as well as possible entry into the mouth or nose.

4. Supervise and evaluate self-application if medication is kept at the bedside and replenish supplies needed for application in resident's bathroom or bedside drawer.

5. Avoid applying excessive amounts of ointment as this can irritate skin.

❧ EVALUATION

Reported relief of skin discomfort, improved condition of skin, skin integrity maintained

MEDICATIONS, SUBCUTANEOUS INJECTION

Subcutaneous (SC) medications are administered by injection into subcutaneous tissue of selected sites that have an adequate amount of healthy tissue for safe injection and absorption. The most common sites used are the upper arm, anterior thigh, and abdomen. Medication that is injected into the subcutaneous tissue is absorbed into the circulation (systemic effect) metabolized by the liver, excreted by the kidneys and are given by this route when residents are unable to take them orally when the drugs may be destroyed by digestive secretions or are inactive when taken orally. The action or absorption is more rapid than the oral route but slower than the intramuscular route as muscle tissue is more vascular than subcutaneous tissue. Medications for injection are available in sterile, one-dose or multiple-dose vials. The maximum amount of solution injected subcutaneously is about 1 ml. Sterile technique is utilized for all subcutaneous injections.

ASSESSMENT

Possible site for adequate subcutaneous tissue, site of last injection, allergies to drugs, age and weight, and general health and circulation status, history of diabetes mellitus or cardiovascular disorders

NURSING DIAGNOSES

Pain, High Risk for Injury; Impaired Tissue Integrity

GOALS

Safe and correct administration of medication via the subcutaneous route

INTERVENTIONS

Equipment/Supplies

- Medication in properly-labeled vial
- Needles of appropriate size of ⅜ to ⅝ inches and appropriate gauge of 24 to 28 depending on solution
- Insulin syringe (U-100) in sterile package or sterile with needle covered
- Sponges with antiseptic
- 1 to 2 ml sterile syringe calibrated in ml or minim or tuberculin syringe without needle
- Biohazard puncture-resistant container for proper disposal

Resident

- Explain purpose of procedure and expected results
- Place in sitting, supine position depending on site to be used and drape to expose area as needed

PROCEDURE

1. Perform medication check with medication sheet, physician written order (before preparation, before taking to resident, before administration to resident).

2. Become familiar with drug action, dose, route, side effects, interactions, expected response using a drug reference.

3. Determine whether to administer or withhold medication based on laboratory test results (blood glucose, urinary glucose/ketones, partial thromboplastin time).

4. Determine appropriate syringe and needle for medication to be administered and site to be used.

5. Perform handwashing.

6. Remove syringe from package, attach needle if packaged separately, maintaining sterile technique.

7. Remove the metal cap or cover on the vial. If a multidose vial is used, cleanse the rubber diaphragm with an antiseptic sponge.

8. Remove needle cover and withdraw the volume of air that is the same as the volume of medication to be withdrawn from the vial, while careful not to touch anything but the syringe barrel and tip of the plunger.

9. Puncture vial diaphragm with the needle and expel the air into the vial above the level of the medication; while holding vial upright and the needle tip covered by the solution with the dominant hand, withdraw the desired amount of medication into the syringe with the dominant hand.

10. Withdraw needle from vial and expel air leaving 0.1 to 0.2 ml to clear needle of the medication during the injection.

11. Place syringe containing the medication with the identifying medication sheet, card or vial.

12. If mixing medication in the same syringe (as in insulins) to avoid giving two injections, check compatibility and withdraw amount of air into the syringe equal to the amount of medication to be withdrawn from the second vial, clean the top of the vial and inject the air into the vial above the level of the medication; change the needle and withdraw the amount of air into the syringe equal to the amount of medication to be withdrawn from the first bottle and follow the procedure of injecting the air and withdrawing the medication as outlined in #9.

13. With the correct amount of medication in the syringe, insert the needle into the second vial and withdraw correct amount of additional medication into the syringe, withdraw the plunge, and allow 0.1 to 0.2 ml of air to enter syringe.

14. Place syringe containing the medication with the identifying medication sheet, card or vial.

15. Take medication to bedside, identify resident by wristband.

16. Palpate and identify site for injection with fingers.

17. Cleanse site with antiseptic sponge.

18. With nondominant hand, grasp a portion of skin between fingers and thumb and insert the needle smoothly and quickly at a 45° angle, or a 90° angle (depending upon the length of the needle used) with the dominant hand.

19. Hold syringe with nondominant hand and aspirate for possible puncture into a blood vessel by noting blood in the syringe. Do not aspirate heparin.

20. Inject medication into the tissue slowly, no faster than 1 ml/4 seconds.

21. Place antiseptic sponge at side of needle, apply slight pressure and withdraw needle.

22. Massage site gently, then wipe site gently. Note: Do not massage site if insulin or heparin is administered.

23. Apply bandaid if needed.

24. Discard syringe, needle and supplies used according to Universal Precautions in a biohazard container.

25. Store medication for future use if appropriate.

26. Wash hands.

❧ PROBLEM-SOLVING ACTIONS

1. Perform assessment required for specific medication, including laboratory tests.

2. Note drug labeling for the route to be used before administering as complications may occur if injected by improper route.

3. Gloves should be worn in those cases where Universal Precautions dictate this measure.

4. Follow drawings on the chart to ensure rotation of sites, and mark site "x" after administration to ensure selection of a new site for the next injection.

5. Use insulin syringe in unit calibration that matches unit dosage on vial.

6. Determine sequence of withdrawing medications from vial when mixing drugs in the same syringe to obtain correct dosage and prevent contamination of a multidose vial.

7. Store parenteral medications in appropriate manner, in medication cart, medication room, refrigerator, room temperature.

8. Sign appropriate forms when administering controlled substances.

9. Administer dosage strength that gives the smallest volume to attain the desired dose.

10. A sufficient amount of subcutaneous tissue may allow for spreading the skin instead of pinching it to administer the medication; a shorter needle (⅝") may require a 90° angle and a larger needle (1-2") a 45° angle for insertion.

✎ EVALUATION

Successful administration of medications via the subcutaneous injection route without incident

MEDICATIONS, SUBLINGUAL/BUCCAL

S ublingual (SL) medications are administered under the tongue, and buccal medications are administered in the upper cheek next to the molars. Both are absorbed through the mucosa into circulation. Sublingual tablets are usually small. The most common drug administered by this route is nitroglycerin which relieves angina pain within 30 seconds to 1 minute. Buccal tablets are larger and some may be absorbed by the pharynx when swallowed with saliva. Clean technique is utilized for sublingual or buccal medication administration.

❧ ASSESSMENT

Chest pain radiating to arm, shoulder, or jaw, history of angina pectoris; other conditions to be treated and drugs used

❧ NURSING DIAGNOSES

Pain

❧ GOALS

Relief of angina pain within 1 minute; safe and correct administration of drug via the sublingual or buccal route

❧ INTERVENTIONS

Equipment/Supplies

- Medication in properly labeled unit dose package
- Medication cup

Resident

- Explain purpose of procedure and expected results
- Place in position of comfort

❧ PROCEDURE

1. Perform medication check with medication sheet, physician written order (before preparation, before taking to resident, before administration to resident).
2. Become familiar with the drug action, dose, route, form, side effects, interactions, expected results using a drug reference.
3. Determine if buccal or sublingual route is to be used for administration.
4. Perform handwashing.
5. Take medication to the resident.
6. Identify the resident by wristband.
7. Remove tablet from package and place it under the tongue or in the upper pouch between cheek and molars.
8. Request the resident to leave tablet in place until it dissolves and not to chew or swallow it as this alters the drug's absorption.
9. Remove medication for future use and store in resident's drawer in medicine cart.
10. Wash hands.

❧ PROBLEM-SOLVING ACTIONS

1. Repeat sublingual nitroglycerin if pain is not relieved in 5 minutes up to 3 tablets within a 15 minute period of time or administer 5 to 10 minutes before activity or as ordered by the physician.

2. Supervise and evaluate self-administration of sublingual nitroglycerin with bottle of medication kept in drawer of bedside table for immediate access by resident.

3. Note expiration date on nitroglycerin as effect of drug is diminished if out-of-date.

4. Remind to hold tablet in place and not to chew or swallow it as this renders it ineffective.

❧ EVALUATION

Reported relief of angina pain, desired results from other medication given via sublingual or buccal route

MEDICATIONS, TRANSDERMAL

Transdermal medications are administered to areas of the skin that are relatively free of hair that facilitate the desired effects of the drug (systemic effect). The most common drug administered by this route is nitroglycerin which provides sustained vasodilation in the prevention and treatment of angina. The drug is available in premeasured adhesive patches in a variety of dosages (2.5 to 15.0 mg) and applied in the frequency ordered by the physician. The drug is absorbed by the skin into the blood stream. Clean technique is utilized for this procedure.

ASSESSMENT

Chest pain radiating to arm, shoulder, or jaw, history of angina attacks

NURSING DIAGNOSES

Pain; High Risk for Impaired Skin Integrity

GOALS

Relief and control of angina; safe and correct administration of the drug via the transdermal route

INTERVENTIONS

Equipment/Supplies

- Medication in properly labeled package
- Adhesive remover, gauze squares
- Warm water, mild soap, towel

Resident

- Explain purpose of procedure and expected results
- Place in sitting or lying position that allows for exposure of area to apply patch

PROCEDURE

1. Perform medication check with medication sheet, physician written order (before preparation, before taking to resident, before administration to resident).
2. Become familiar with the drug action, dose, route, form, side effects, interactions, expected results using a drug reference.
3. Perform handwashing.
4. Take medication to the bedside and identify resident by wristband.
5. Remove old patch and cleanse area of tape with tape remover and gently wash with warm water and mild soap and pat dry.
6. Remove the patch from the package, peel off the cover on the side of the patch that will be attached to the skin.
7. Apply the patch to the skin, apply gentle pressure to seal the edges and ensure that the medication will have contact with the skin.
8. Request the resident to leave the patch in place, to avoid picking at it or touching it and to avoid getting it wet when bathing.
9. Wash hands.

❧ PROBLEM-SOLVING ACTIONS

1. Rotate sites of application to prevent skin irritation.

2. Avoid touching medication side of patch as the medication will be absorbed by the skin on the fingers administering a dose of the medication to the nurse.

3. Usual frequency of application of transdermal patch is every 24 hours and should be applied at same time of day to ensure continuity of dosage.

❧ EVALUATION

Absence or control of angina attacks reported, skin integrity maintained at sites of application

MEDICATIONS, VAGINAL SUPPOSITORY/CREAM

*V*aginal suppository (SUPP) or cream are medications that are inserted into the vagina to treat infections with antimicrobials or vaginal atrophy with hormones (local effect). The suppository is a cone or cylinder shape in a firm base and is administered with an applicator or gloved finger. The cream is a soft base and is administered with a plunger applicator. Both forms dissolve at body temperature. Clean technique is utilized for vaginal medication administration.

ASSESSMENT

Discharge or odor from vagina; itching or discomfort in genital area; history of gynecologic disorder; age post-menopausal

NURSING DIAGNOSES

High Risk for Infection; Impaired Tissue Integrity (Secretions)

GOALS

Maintenance of vaginal mucosa, absence or control of vaginal infection and genitalia discomfort

INTERVENTIONS

Equipment/Supplies

- Medication in proper form and labeling in package or tube
- Plunger application or insertion device
- Disposable gloves
- Water-soluble lubricant
- Bed protector
- Warm water, mild soap, towel
- Light source

Resident

- Explain purpose of procedure and expected results
- Place light source directed at perineum
- Place in supine position with knees flexed and drape to expose genitalia

PROCEDURE

1. Perform medication check with medication sheet, physician written order (before preparation, before taking to resident, before administration to resident).
2. Become familiar with the drug action, dose, route, form, side effects, interactions, expected results using the drug reference.
3. Determine which form is to be administered and type of applicator to use.
4. Perform handwashing.
5. Take medication and supplies to the bedside.
6. Identify resident by wristband.
7. Place bed protector under buttocks.
8. Cleanse perineum with warm water and mild soap, pat dry.

9. Put disposable gloves on.

10. Remove suppository from package, and place in applicator device if used, fill calibrated plunger applicator by attaching it to the tube and squeezing the desired amount to be instilled.

11. Lubricate the applicator or finger if used to insert suppository or instill cream.

12. With nondominant hand, separate labia to expose vaginal orifice and with dominant hand holding the applicator or index finger, insert the suppository or cream with the full length of the applicator or finger (about 2 to 3 inches).

13. Remove finger or applicator after inserting or instilling the medication by pushing the plunger into the barrel of the applicator or leaving the suppository in the vagina.

14. Discard applicator or wash with soap and water if reusable and store with medication.

15. Remove gloves and discard properly with other used articles.

16. Request resident to remain in supine position for 30 minutes and apply a perineal pad if needed to prevent staining.

17. Wash hands.

❧ PROBLEM-SOLVING ACTIONS

1. Administer vaginal medication following bathing to eliminate need for perineal care and cleansing before procedure.

2. Place suppository in wrapper under cold running water or in refrigerator if softened.

3. Remove paper covering from suppository.

4. Insert the finger or applicator along the posterior wall of the vagina since this is longer than the anterior wall because of cervical protrusion toward the upper portion of the vaginal wall.

5. Dispersement of the medication will be enhanced if resident remains in the supine position as the vagina has no sphincter muscle to hold the medication.

6. Self-administration of the medications may be preferred and allowed (if possible) if resident is supervised and evaluated for correct technique and desired results.

❧ EVALUATION

Controlled odor and perineal discomfort relief; successful elimination of vaginal infection or symptoms caused by vaginal atrophic condition

UNIT VI

INTRAVENOUS THERAPY

- Infusion Control Device

- Intravenous Fluid Management

- Medications, Intravenous Infusion

- Venipuncture for Intravenous Therapy, Butterfly/Angiocatheter

INFUSION CONTROL DEVICE

Infusion control devices regulate the flow of intravenous (IV) fluids. They ensure the accuracy of the flow rate in the delivery of a specific amount of fluid over a specific period of time. The type of device (gravity controller or infusion pump) is determined by the type of fluid and the frequency of administration. They can be volumetric and ensure the delivery at a constant volume (ml/hour) for long-term administration or nonvolumetric and deliver the fluid at a constant drop rate (gtt/minute) for short-term administration (such as for medications). The gravity controller operates and regulates flow automatically and includes alarms to warn of failures such as an empty container, tubing obstruction, or change in rate. The infusion pump operates by exerting pressure to infuse the fluid such as in a cassette pump. The manufacturer's information and directions accompanies each device.

ASSESSMENT

Reason for use of infusion control device, type of device and therapy, dosage or amounts ordered, frequency of infusion, patency of infusion set

NURSING DIAGNOSES

Anxiety; High Risk for Injury

GOAL

Correct use and operation of infusion control device

INTERVENTIONS

Equipment/Supplies

- Appropriate infusion device for type of therapy
- Appropriate tubing and set up for the selected infusion device
- IV pole

Resident

- Explain the purpose of procedure and expected results
- Place in position of comfort with the intravenous infusion and device within proper proximity

PROCEDURE

1. Perform handwashing.
2. Become familiar with the type of device and reason for infusion, frequency, amount and rate of infusion.
3. Assemble supplies to prepare for intravenous infusion, infusion pump and correct infusion set.
4. Attach the pump to the IV pole and hang the solution with tubing clamped and drip chamber ⅓ full and positioned 6-12 inches above the pump.
5. Prepare and administer fluids via the gravity controller:
   a. Rotate the drip chamber to ensure that the fluid touches all sides.

b. Prime the tubing and clamp.

c. Place the drop sensor above the level of fluid in the drip chamber and lower than the drop port.

d. Insert the tubing and close the door of the controller, connect to the venipuncture cannula, then open the clamp controlling the flow.

e. Plug in the machine and set the dials to infusion rate and volume, turn the machine on and press the button to start.

6. Prepare and administer fluids via the cassette-type infusion pump:

a. Invert the cassette with flat side facing operator, unclamp and allow the solution to fill the entire tubing.

b. Clamp tubing, connect tubing to the venipuncture cannula and turn the device on.

c. Rotate the load knob counter clockwise, press key to silence alarm.

d. Turn door lock and press latch to open door, align holes in the cassette with the pins in the cassette house, close door and latch to lock.

e. Rotate knob clockwise to IN, unclamp tubing and set to select alarm threshold, press key to clear.

f. Enter desired volume, rate, and press key to begin the infusion.

7. Tape all connections to prevent leakage or dislodgement.

8. Provide site care, tubing change, and monitoring of rate and volume (see Intravenous Fluid Management for complete care procedures).

❧ PROBLEM-SOLVING ACTIONS

1. Monitor pump or controller device for rate and volume, site for complications, tubing for patency, I&O for fluid imbalance every 4-8 hours.

2. Set up and operation can vary with devices; follow instructions furnished by manufacturer for specific device.

3. Check alarm systems on the device used, familiarize the resident with the sound and what is means to allay anxiety.

4. Infusion devices can be utilized when administering fluids via other routes such as right atrial catheters for total parenteral nutrition as well as other fluids.

5. Small volume disposable pumps are available for one dose IV administration; some are reusable for administration of a pre-set rate of medication via heparin lock.

❧ EVALUATION

Safe and accurate maintenance of rate and volume intravenous infusion via infusion device

INTRAVENOUS FLUID MANAGEMENT

The management of intravenous (IV) administration includes the procedures performed to ensure safe and correct peripheral infusion of fluid therapy. The varied procedures done are the preparation of the IV solution and set up, IV site care and monitoring, tubing and solution change, calculation and regulation of the flow rate, and discontinuation of the infusion and removal of the cannula. The venipuncture and IV infusion procedures to administer IV fluids are outlined and detailed in separate procedures. Solutions and set ups are selected to reflect the type of IV solution container, and the rate and type of infusion to be administered and prepared prior to the venipuncture. Solutions are available in bottles or bags containing 500 ml or 1000 ml amounts for routine IVs with set ups that deliver rates 60 gtts/ml (microdrip) or 10, 15, 220 gtts/ml (macrodrip). IV site care and tubing/solution is ongoing as long as therapy continues and involves dressing change every 24 hours, tubing change every 48 hours, and solution change every 24 hours or less, as well as monitoring for infiltration and infection at the insertion site. The flow rate regulation involves the calculation of the rate based on the drip rate of the administration set and hourly assessment to ensure that the amount and rate of fluid infused is correct. This includes a flow rate to keep the vein open (KVO) for infusions of fluid or medications. The discontinuation of the IV is performed at the conclusion of the IV therapy and involves the removal of the cannula and dressing application to the site. Those procedures that involve sterile supplies and the IV site should be performed utilizing sterile technique.

ASSESSMENT

Type, length of time, and reason for therapy, type of fluid, amount, flow rate in ml/hour and drop rate in gtt/minute, type of administration set up and solution container, site of venipuncture and patency, need for site care and solution/tubing change, vital signs, I&O balance

NURSING DIAGNOSES

High Risk for Fluid Deficit or Excess; High Risk for Infection; Anxiety; High Risk for Impaired Tissue Integrity

GOAL

Effective management and maintenance of intravenous fluid therapy without complications

INTERVENTIONS

Equipment/Supplies

- Bag or bottle of fluid to be infused
- Correct administration set
- IV pole
- Sterile dressings, tape, antiseptic swabs
- Antiseptic ointment
- Disposable gloves
- Band aid

Resident

- Explain the purpose of procedure and expected results
- Place in position of comfort with infusion site exposed

❧ PROCEDURE

1. Perform handwashing.

2. Become familiar with the infusion site used, infusion patency, amount of solution and drop rate, administration set needed, renal or cardiac condition, hematology or bleeding disorders, and use of an infusion control device.

3. Assemble the supplies needed to perform specific procedures on a flat clean surface within close proximity to the resident; include a controller or pump if used.

4. Prepare the solution/set up for IV administration:
   a. Examine the bottle or bag of solution for cracks, leaks, cloudiness or particles, expiration date; open administration set box and check for correct tubing and drip system, that tips are covered and clamps are on the tubing.
   b. Label the bag or bottle and IV line with the date that it was placed into use.
   c. Remove the cover or cap from the spike on the set and the cap from the port on the bag or if a bottle is used, remove the metal cap and inner cover; insert the spike from the set into the port on the bag or the larger hole in the rubber stopper on the bottle after cleansing with an antiseptic swab.
   d. Invert the bag or bottle and hang on the pole 24 inches above the IV site.
   e. Squeeze the drip chamber and allow the fluid to flow until it is ½ full while the tubing is clamped.
   f. Remove the cap from the tubing end and unclamp the tubing to allow the fluid to flow through and expel the air.
   g. Remove any remaining air bubbles in the tubing and connect to the cannula in place or reclamp and cap the end and perform venipuncture (see Venipuncture for Intravenous Therapy, Butterfly/ Angiocatheter).
   h. Adjust the drop and volume rate according to amount and rate of infusion or insert tubing into the control device and set for the amount/hour (see Infusion Control Device).

5. Perform IV line and site maintenance:
   a. Assess tubing for kinking and patency, drop rate, volume being infused every hour and adjust as needed; maintain the drip chamber ½ full.
   b. Assess site for needle displacement, infiltration, and need for dressing change.
   c. Remove immobilized arm from armboard every 2-4 hours and carefully exercise and note any stiffness.
   d. Change dressing if soiled or wet with sterile gauze square and retape cannula and tubing in place.
   e. Change IV bag or bottle of fluid at least every 24 hours by clamping the tubing, removing the cap from the new container port, prepare top of the container, removing the spike from the empty container and inserting it into the port or top of the new container; rehang, unclamp the tubing and readjust the gtt or ml rate.
   f. Change the administration set at least every 48 hours by removing the tubing from the box, clamping with the cover in place on the spike, removing the old tubing from the container and then inserting the spike into the port or top of the container while the fluid remaining in the old tubing continues to flow into the cannula; rehang the container, prime the tubing and replace cap on the end removing the old tubing from the cannula; and cover from the new tubing and inserting it into the cannula; unclamp the tubing and readjust the gtt or ml rate.
   g. Dispose of all used supplies according to universal precautions.

6. Calculate and regulate the flow rate:
   a. Note the gtt/ml rate on the administration set used and total volume of fluid and time to be administered.
   b. Using a formula, ratio-proportion, or dimensional analysis method, calculate the desired drip rate to administer the correct amount over a period of time.
   c. Note the number of drops into the chamber and time for 1 minute with a watch.
   d. Adjust the clamp and count the drops for 1 minute, readjust the clamp as needed until the correct drop rate is achieved.
   e. Assess flow rate and volume every hour and adjust as needed.
   f. Adjust to a rate to keep the vein open (KVO) if future infusions expected.

7. Discontinue the IV therapy:
   a. Clamp the tubing.
   b. Carefully remove the tape and dressing at the insertion site while holding the cannula in place and pulling the tape toward the insertion site.

   c. Hold a sterile gauze over the insertion site with the nondominant hand and gently but firmly remove the cannula with one movement with the dominant hand, check the angiocatheter to be sure that the cannula is intact.

   d. Apply pressure to the site until the bleeding stops.

   e. Apply and tape a small bandage to the site.

   f. Dispose of all used supplies according to universal precautions.

8. Place in a position of comfort following IV care procedures.

❧ PROBLEM-SOLVING ACTIONS

1. Tape all IV connections to prevent displacement or leakage if appropriate.

2. Assess site for pain, redness or other color change, edema, pain and, if present, discontinue and restart at a different site.

3. A chart that offers gtts/min to infuse a given amount over a period of time is usually made available for the different set ups eliminating the need for calculations.

4. I&O monitoring should be done every 4-8 hours on all residents receiving IV fluids.

5. Gowns can be changed by removing the sleeves from the arms first with the sleeve on the arm receiving the IV left on the tubing, removing the container from the pole and slipping it through the sleeve and inserting it into the sleeve of the clean gown that will be slipped on the IV arm; replace the container on the pole and continue to put the other sleeve of the gown on the other arm.

6. Correct causes of rates that are too fast or too slow by noting any position changes, blood pressure changes, bending arm or clamp manipulation, dangling or kinking in tubing, obstruction of cannula, and other problems.

7. Never increase the rate if the fluid amount refused is less than desired, readjust to the appropriate rate instead.

❧ EVALUATION

IV therapy and daily management performed with safety and accuracy, patent IV infusion, correct rate, volume, and time calculations and administration, insertion site free of untoward effects of therapy

MEDICATIONS, INTRAVENOUS INFUSION

Intravenous medications are administered to provide a more rapid effect and a more effective absorption than other parenteral routes. IV medications can be administered continuously over a long period via a secondary infusion utilizing a measured container device, piggyback container, or a single IV infusion such as a bolus via the IV line or heparin lock device. The administration of IV medications requires correct calculations for flow rate, time, and dilutions in order to control the rapidity with which the drug reaches the circulation. Another important consideration is the risk of mixing incompatible drugs in the IV tubing, a complication that can be prevented by avoiding the administration of more than one drug unless the tubing is cleared with water or saline injection prior to the medication infusion. Sterile technique is utilized for IV medication administration.

❧ ASSESSMENT

Drug allergies, condition/illness being treated, method, time, and frequency of administration, compatibility of drugs, type of IV solution and administration set used, patency of line or device

❧ NURSING DIAGNOSES

High Risk for Infection; High Risk for Injury; Anxiety

❧ GOAL

Safe and correct administration of medications via the IV route

❧ INTERVENTIONS

Equipment/Supplies

- IV administration set with Y injection ports
- IV administration set for piggyback or volume control device to connect to the main line
- Heparin flush for heparin lock device
- Sterile normal saline or water in syringe with needle connected

- Medications to be injected, added to a solution, or already prepared in solution
- Antiseptic swabs

- Disposable gloves

Resident

- Explain purpose of procedure and expected results
- Place in position of comfort with IV site and line exposed

❧ PROCEDURE

1. Perform medications check with medication sheet, physician written order.
2. Become familiar with drug action, dose, side effects, compatibilities, time and rate of infusion, expected response.
3. Perform handwashing.

4. Assemble the necessary supplies and medication based on the type of administration on a clean surface; identify resident by wrist band or other method.

5. Prepare and add medication to an IV solution for continuous administration:
   a. Draw up the accurate dosage of medications from an ampule or vial into a sterile syringe with a needle attached or prepare by unit dose in a syringe.
   b. Change the needle and cleanse the injection port or stopper on the bag or bottle of solution with an antiseptic swab.
   c. Inject the medication into the solution (500 ml, 1000 ml), remove the empty syringe.
   d. Gently move the container back and forth to evenly distribute the medication in the solution.
   e. Hang the solution container and connect the set up tubing to the cannula (see Intravenous Fluid Management for procedures to prepare the set up and solution).
   f. Unclamp the tubing and adjust the rate to administer the correct amount of solution and correct dosage of medication, usually slowly over 8-10 hours.
   g. Record the drug name, dose, rate, date, and time drug added on the container.

6. Prepare and administer a bolus injection:
   a. Withdraw the correct dosage properly diluted into a sterile syringe with a needle attached.
   b. Change the needle and prepare the skin site for venipuncture.
   c. Perform venipuncture (see Venipuncture for Intravenous Therapy) with the needle and syringe of medication.
   d. Release the tourniquet and slowly inject the medication over a period of time, not less than 1 minute with 3-5 minutes preferred, note response from resident during the procedure.
   e. Remove the needle and apply pressure to the site until bleeding stops, apply a bandaid.
   f. Bolus can be injected into an injection port close to the cannula site, following cleansing with an antiseptic swab, by inserting the needle into the port, pinching the tubing and withdrawing the syringe plunger for a blood return, then releasing the tubing and slowly injecting the medication over 3-5 minutes; then withdrawing the needle and empty syringe and noting any side effects during and after the injection.
   g. Flush the line with normal saline before and after the injection if the medication is not compatible with the IV infusion.
   h. Readjust the flow rate on the primary IV following the bolus injection through the port.

7. Prepare and administer medications via a heparin lock device:
   a. Withdraw the medication in the correct amount and dilution into a sterile syringe with a needle attached.
   b. Cleanse the self sealing diaphragm of the device with an antiseptic swab and flush the device with sterile normal saline solution in a cartridge or prepare in a sterile syringe and needle.
   c. Replace the needle on the syringe of medication and inject into the diaphragm on the device over 3-5 minutes and reflush with heparin solution (100 U/1 ml) to maintain patency.
   d. Flush the device with normal saline before and after the medication is injected if the medication is not compatible with the heparin.

8. Prepare and administer medications via measured container:
   a. Remove the volume control set from the container and the guard from the spike and close the clamps on the container.
   b. Insert spike into the solution container and hang on a pole.
   c. Open the clamps on the air vent and on the lower IV tubing and position it up near the volume control chamber, clamp the tubing.
   d. Allow the fluid chamber to fill with 30 ml of the solution by opening the upper clamp, reclamp and squeeze the drip chamber until it is ½ full.
   e. Open the lower clamp and prime the tubing, reclamp.
   f. Depending on the use of a primary or secondary line, insert an adapter into the cannula hub or attach a needle to the adapter on the volume control set respectively, cleanse the injection port with an antiseptic swab and insert the needle, secure the connections with tape.
   g. Cleanse the injection port on the volume control container and inject the medication that has been prepared in a sterile syringe with a needle attached.
   h. Unclamp the upper tubing and fill the chamber with the desired amount of fluid, reclamp and gently mix by rotating the device.

   i. Clamp the tubing to the existing IV infusion or maintain at lowest possible drop rate, open the lower clamp on the device and adjust the drop rate to administer the correct volume and dosage of the medication.

   j. At the conclusion of the medication infusion, open the upper clamp and allow 10 ml of solution to flow into the device and tubing to flush the chamber and line.

   k. If the device is used as a secondary line, clamp the lower tubing and readjust the flow rate of the primary line; if the device is used as a primary line, clamp the lower tubing, allow the chamber to fill to the desired amount and begin the infusion for intermittent administration without the administration of a continuous IV infusion.

9. Prepare and administer medications via piggyback:
   a. If the container of solution is not premixed with medication, withdraw the medication into a sterile syringe with a needle attached and inject into the port after it has been cleansed with an antiseptic swab.
   b. Gently move back and forth to mix the solutions.
   c. Remove the secondary administration set from the container and connect to the administration port the container of fluid.
   d. Prime the tubing and attach a needle to it, cleanse the Y port on the primary line and insert the needle into it, secure the connection with tape.
   e. Adjust the rate and allow the secondary line to flow until empty.
   f. When the piggyback container is empty, open the clamp on the primary line and readjust the drop rate as needed for the primary IV infusion.
   g. If an infusion device is used to administer the secondary line, insert the line proximal to the device, clamp the primary line and reset the device for the desired flow rate of the piggyback administration; upon completion, unclamp the primary line and readjust the flow rate for the primary infusion.

10. Dispose of all used articles and supplies according to Universal Precautions.

11. Note response to the medication during and after administration.

❧ PROBLEM-SOLVING ACTIONS

1. Be aware that complications from IV administration of medications include phlebitis and thrombophlebitis, infiltration, air embolism, speed shock, and circulatory overload and assess for these untoward effects.

2. Check the medications to be sure that they can be administered over long or short periods of time for best response to the therapy.

3. If possible, an infusion pump should be used to administer the correct dosage in the correct time frame.

4. If adding a drug to a solution already running, clamp and inject the medication into the port, rotate to mix, unclamp and readjust the drop rate.

5. Be aware of drug reactions or sensitivities during the infusion.

❧ EVALUATION

IV medications administered safely and accurately via the appropriate route and method at dosage and frequency ordered; no complications or untoward effects present

VENIPUNCTURE FOR INTRAVENOUS THERAPY, BUTTERFLY/ANGIOCATHETER

*V*enipuncture for intravenous (IV) therapy is the technique of introducing a cannula into a peripheral vein for continuous or intermittent administration of fluids and to maintain an open vein to avoid the necessity of repeated punctures. It is a commonly used route used to provide short-term fluid and nutritional needs as well as to administer medications, blood, and blood products. Intravenous fluids that are used include dextrose in water or saline solutions, normal saline solutions, and electrolyte solutions. The venipuncture procedure involves the selection of an appropriate venous site and proper type, length, and gauge of a device or cannula (butterfly steel needle or plastic catheter) to be inserted into the vein. Strict sterile technique is utilized for all aspects of the procedure of venipuncture, the initial step in performing intravenous therapy. Associated intravenous therapy procedures are outlined in this section and should follow or be performed in conjunction with venipuncture.

ASSESSMENT

Reason for and type of fluids to be administered, type and size of needle, duration of the IV, condition of the veins and skin at most distal sites on the hands and forearms, need for site immobilization, I&O

NURSING DIAGNOSES

Anxiety; High Risk for Fluid Volume Deficit or Excess; High Risk for Infection; High Risk for Impaired Skin Integrity; Altered Nutrition: Less Than Body Requirements; High Risk for Injury

GOAL

Safe and correct performance of venipuncture for IV therapy using the appropriate equipment

INTERVENTIONS

Equipment/Supplies

- Butterfly or angiocatheter device
- Tourniquet
- Antiseptic swabs, ointment
- Sterile dressing, transparent film dressing
- Armboard or other restraint
- Tape
- Disposable gloves

Resident

- Explain the purpose of procedure and expected results
- Place in low-Fowler's position with arm and hand exposed

PROCEDURE

1. Perform handwashing.
2. Become familiar with the reason for the venipuncture and the cannula and site to be used if IV therapy is continuous or intermittent.
3. Select the superficial vein site on the back of the hand or forearm and note size, patency, and proneness to collapse.
4. Place a protective pad under the hand or arm.

5. Put on disposable gloves.

6. Shave the area if necessary.

7. Place the tourniquet above the site and palpate the distended vein to be used.

8. Release the tourniquet after the desirable vein is palpated and selected.

9. Cleanse the site with the antiseptic swabs from the center outward and reapply the tourniquet between the site and the heart with a loop tie.

10. Perform venipuncture with a butterfly cannula:
    a. Prepare the butterfly cannula by attaching it to the primed tubing of the administration set.
    b. Place the thumb of the nondominant hand to the side and 1 inch distal to the vein insertion site and pull skin taut.
    c. With the dominant hand, hold the needle with the bevel side up and parallel to the vein at a 45-degree angle.
    d. Insert the needle holding the wings between the thumb and forefinger and lower to a 10-degree angle, note a blood return and advance the needle to the hilt.
    e. Release the tourniquet, slip a piece of tape under the hilt and allow the ends to cover the open wings, position the tape over the hilt of the needle to secure it in the vein.
    f. Secure the tubing to the arm, unclamp and start infusion (see Intravenous Fluid Management for administration and care procedures).

11. Perform venipuncture with an angiocatheter:
    a. Follow the same procedure outlined above for the butterfly cannula up to the point of advancing the device into the vein.
    b. Advance the catheter by holding the catheter hub with the nondominant hand and gently moving the catheter into the vein for the full length with the dominant hand following insertion into the vein.
    c. Withdraw the needle from the plastic catheter sheath that is left in the vein, connect the hub to the tubing and note a blood return in the backflow chamber.
    d. Unclamp the tubing and allow the infusion to begin.
    e. Apply an antiseptic ointment to the site and cover with a sterile gauge or transparent dressing and tape leaving the hub connection site free of the dressings.
    f. Secure the tubing to the arm and write the date, size and type of device (see Intravenous Fluid Management for administration and care procedures).

12. Remove gloves and discard with other used supplies according to universal precautions.

13. If needed, immobilize the arm in an armboard in a comfortable position.

❧ PROBLEM-SOLVING ACTIONS

1. Veins that are found to be difficult to cannulate can be made more accessible by applying warm compresses to the site or lowering the arm below the heart level.

2. Change cannula according to agency policy and use the smallest gauge device possible.

3. Infiltration that occurs when the tubing is unclamped requires removal of the device and another site chosen for venipuncture using a new device and supplies.

4. If there is no blood return after inserting the device into the vein, pull it back and rotate to remove the possibility of the bevel resting against the wall of the vein, or pinch the tubing, or lower the fluid bag below the site level; remove the device and recannulate if these do not establish venous access.

5. Assessment of the skin site for redness, pain indicating infection and I&O indicating a fluid imbalance should be done every 4-8 hours during IV therapy.

6. If Hep Lock cannula insertion into a vein for intermittent IV administration is to be performed, follow the same procedure as for the butterfly device except attach a syringe and needle to the hub instead of the administration tubing and test for placement by the injection of 2 ml saline into the device and heparin to maintain patency of device.

❧ EVALUATION

Safe and proper insertion of a butterfly/angiocatheter device performed with patency established

UNIT VII

NEUROLOGIC PROCEDURES

- Neurologic Checks
- Seizure Precautions
- Transcutaneous Electrical Nerve Stimulation (TENS)

NEUROLOGIC CHECKS

Neurologic checks are a combination of objective observations and measurements done to evaluate neurologic status that includes consciousness, orientation, pupillary changes, neuromuscular function and neurosensory perception. The results of the checks assist to determine nervous system damage and/or deterioration.

❧ ASSESSMENT

Level of consciousness, mental status, vital signs, sensory and motor responses, history of stroke and presence of paralysis, intracranial disorders, neuromuscular disorders

❧ NURSING DIAGNOSES

Impaired Physical Mobility; High Risk for Trauma; Altered Thought Processes, Sensory/Perceptual Alterations

❧ GOALS

Identification of changes indicating progressive improvement or deterioration in neurologic status, correct and thorough neurologic checks

❧ INTERVENTIONS

Equipment/Supplies

- Penlight
- Thermometer, sphygmomanometer, stethoscope
- Chart to check pupil size
- Glasgow Coma Scale to score function

Resident

- Explain purpose of procedure and reason based on ability to understand

❧ PROCEDURE

1. Perform handwashing.
2. Become familiar with general physical assessment and history of neurologic disorders and conditions affecting mental status.
3. Assess vital signs, temperature, pulse, respirations, and blood pressure.
4. Check orientation via verbal responses to questions regarding name, place, person, date, time, and events; attention span, mood, affect, and behavior.
5. Check ability to respond to verbal commands, raise arm, close eyes, move in bed.
6. Check response to tactile stimuli, squeeze hand, apply pressure to arm or leg on both sides of body.
7. Check eyes for size and shape and ability to open and close; note symmetry of both eyes, compare pupil size to chart and equality.
8. Use penlight to check response of pupils to light, direct light from outer to inner aspect of eye and note constriction, dilation when the light is removed; compare both eyes for equality, constriction and dilation (PERL).

9. Check eye movement by noting ability to follow finger with eyes in all directions, ability to focus on finger while moving it towards the nose.

10. Check ability to open and close eye lids, presence of ptosis of lid.

11. Check eye movements on unconscious resident by moving the head to the side with eyes open and note that eye will move in opposite direction of the rotation (doll's eyes) and by moving head up or down and note that the eye movement will be in the opposite direction.

12. Check grip of hand and ability to squeeze a hand and compare strength in both hands.

13. Check strength of both arms and legs by having resident close eyes and extend arms out in front with palms up and raise legs one at a time and push down on them; arms that drift down indicate muscle weakness.

14. Note any spontaneous movement if resident is unconscious to check motor strength or note any resistance to range of motion exercises.

15. Note muscle tone, motor gait, tremor, membranes or tingling in extremities.

❧ PROBLEM-SOLVING ACTIONS

1. Note deterioration of neurologic status by changes in responses to painful stimuli, posturing and presence of flexion and extension of body parts.

2. Perform deep reflex assessment and cranial nerve evaluation if indicated.

3. Use Glasgow Coma Scale to determine level of consciousness.

4. Frequency of checks is every 15 minutes for 1 hour, every 30 minutes for next hour, every 60 minutes for remaining hours for a total of 72 hours.

❧ EVALUATION

Neurologic checks performed correctly and noted at frequency indicated by resident's condition with changes reported

SEIZURE PRECAUTIONS

Seizure precautions are measures taken to protect the resident from injury resulting from changes in consciousness. Causes of seizures range from a history of seizure activity (epilepsy) to conditions that may precipitate seizure activity such as noncompliance in medication administration.

ASSESSMENT

Anticonvulsant being taken, history of seizure activity and type of seizures (partial or generalized) and characteristics if known (motor, somatosensory, autonomic, psychic)

NURSING DIAGNOSES

High Risk for Injury; High Risk for Ineffective Breathing Pattern; Altered Thought Processes

GOAL

Prevention of injury during seizure activity

INTERVENTIONS

Equipment/Supplies

- Blankets for padding
- Oral airway
- Suction equipment if needed (machine and catheter)
- Bite stick

Resident

- Explain purpose of procedure and preventive actions taken and rationale for action

PROCEDURE

1. Perform handwashing.
2. Become familiar with cause and type of previous seizure activity, anticonvulsant being administered to treat condition.
3. Pad sides (siderails) and top of bed, sides and back of wheelchair with blankets and secure them with safety pins.
4. Place the suction equipment within reach and set up ready for use.
5. Tape the bite stick in a plastic bag to head of bed.
6. Place an airway in a plastic bag on bedside table or tape to the head of the bed.
7. If seizure occurs when standing, ease patient to floor being careful to protect head.
8. Avoid restricting movement of the resident during the seizure and remain with the resident until seizure has ended; maintain a patent airway.
9. If an aura is experienced, assist to bed with siderails up and remain with resident.
10. At conclusion of the seizure, allow the resident to sleep and/or remain in bed until ready to resume activity.

❧ PROBLEM-SOLVING ACTIONS

1. If possible, note type of aura and where seizure originates.
2. Note atonic, clonic and tonic type and length of time and any other manifestations of the seizure.
3. Ensure that anticonvulsant medications are administered correctly and check for therapeutic level of drug if laboratory testing done.
4. Avoid use of oral thermometer for monitoring temperature to prevent biting it if a seizure should occur.

❧ EVALUATION

Seizure activity minimized, absence of injury during seizure

TRANSCUTANEOUS ELECTRICAL NERVE STIMULATION (TENS)

Transcutaneous electrical nerve stimulation is a procedure that provides electrical impulses to a painful area using an electrical-powered device. This electrical current blocks the transmission of pain impulses to the brain. Its general use is restricted to clients with chronic pain in order to reduce the need for analgesic therapy. The portable device allows the client to adjust the intensity and rate of the stimulation based on the intensity, duration, and frequency of the pain being experienced. Lead wires connected to the device and to the electrodes on the skin at the area to be treated provide the source and pathway for the electric current.

ASSESSMENT

Pain and its characteristics, area to be treated, history of disorders causing chronic pain, such as arthritis or presence of pacemaker that would disallow use of TENS

NURSING DIAGNOSES

Chronic Pain; High Risk for Impaired Skin Integrity

GOALS

Relief of pain, skin integrity maintained, correct application and use of TENS

INTERVENTIONS

Equipment/Supplies

- Transcutaneous electrical nerve stimulator
- Charged battery pack and battery recharger
- Electrodes (reusable or disposable) and pin connectors
- Lead wires
- Electrode gel and tape if needed
- Alcohol sponges

Resident

- Explain purpose of procedure and expected results
- Place in position of comfort with area to be treated exposed and properly draped

PROCEDURE

1. Perform handwashing.
2. Become familiar with cause, location, severity and frequency of pain and use of analgesics to control pain; past effectiveness of TENS.
3. Select proper size and type of electrodes based on area to be treated and if they are to be used just once or stay on for future use.
4. Check battery on device by turning on the controls and noting blinking lights.
5. Connect lead wires into the stimulator at the appropriate jacks.
6. Set amplitude, rate, width, and modulation controls at desired regulation of device.
7. Identify resident by wristband.

8. Clean skin of area with alcohol sponge and allow to dry.

9. Plug lead wires into the appropriate end of the electrode(s).

10. Peel electrode from the liners and moisten with tap water, wait for a minute or until it becomes sticky; if prepared electrode is not used, apply electrode gel to the electrode bottom.

11. Apply the sticky electrode to the skin and press firmly, if electrode gel is used, place electrode on skin and tape around the edges to ensure that they are firmly attached.

12. Loop the wires and tape to the back of the electrodes if needed.

13. Turn device on and time the procedure during the presence of a tingling sensation.

14. Turn device off when procedure completed and remove lead wires if electrode is to remain for future treatments or remove electrode by carefully and gently peeling it off.

15. Cleanse sites with warm water and mild soap, pat dry.

16. Leave the resident in comfortable position.

17. Place the rechargeable battery into the charger that is plugged into an outlet and replace battery pack when needed.

≥ PROBLEM-SOLVING ACTIONS

1. Clip or shave hair at treatment sites if needed to prevent pulling when removing electrodes.

2. Electrodes may be returned to liners if they are reusable.

3. It is advisable to maintain the device in off position when not in use.

4. Changing the site of the electrodes is permissible, but device must be turned off; incorrect placement will render the treatment ineffective.

5. Improper setting of the controls will prevent optimal effect from the treatment, settings that are high will increase the pain and low settings will prevent pain relief.

6. Electrodes that are left in place should be removed and reapplied daily to allow for skin assessment and care.

7. Adjust the controls according to the resident's tolerance; it may be necessary to turn the device on after application of the electrodes with a gradual adjustment of the controls until optimal tolerance and effect is reached.

8. Alternate sites should be assessed and utilized if application of the electrodes is not possible at the site of pain (as near to pain site as possible and between brain and area).

9. Integrate TENS use with other pain relief measures.

≥ EVALUATION

Pain controlled or relieved, absence of redness, irritation, or breaks in skin at treatment site

UNIT VIII

CARDIOVASCULAR PROCEDURES

- Ace Elastic Bandages
- Antiembolism Hose
- Holter Monitor
- Permanent Pacemaker
- Right Atrial Catheter Management

ACE ELASTIC BANDAGE

Elastic bandages are rolled bandages made of a firm, flexible material and applied to an extremity. They promote venous return, prevent the pooling of blood in an extremity, immobilize a joint or traumatized part to prevent swelling, or secure dressings applied following surgery/treatment of a lesion or ulcer of the extremity. The spiral turn is the technique most commonly used to apply this bandage to an arm or leg.

❧ ASSESSMENT

Body part to be wrapped, presence of varicose vein surgery, leg ulcer, splint, need for joint immobilization, history of impaired peripheral circulation

❧ NURSING DIAGNOSES

Pain; High Risk for Peripheral Neurovascular Dysfunction; Impaired Physical Mobility

❧ GOALS

Relief of discomfort; peripheral circulation within baseline parameters; correct monitoring and application of elastic bandage

❧ INTERVENTIONS

Equipment/Supplies

- Elastic bandage roll in 3, 4, 6 inch widths and 4, 6 foot lengths depending on need
- Sterile gauze bandage, if needed, for skin trauma or to dress surgical incisions
- Clips or safety pin to secure end of bandage

Resident

- Explain purpose of procedure and expected results
- Place in position of comfort with extremity to be bandaged exposed

❧ PROCEDURE

1. Perform handwashing.
2. Become observant of baseline peripheral pulses and skin color and temperature to serve as a comparison; physician order for area to wrapped and duration, whether continuous or intermittent.
3. Select proper size of bandage for area to be wrapped and take to bedside.
4. Identify resident by wristband.
5. Elevate and support extremity for a period of time to allow for venous return before applying the bandage.
6. With the roll held in the dominant hand and facing upward, grasp the end of the roll with the nondominant hand and, beginning with the distal part of the extremity, perform two circular turns to anchor the end around the part.
7. Continue to wrap toward the proximal part by spiral turns with an overlap of the previous turn of about ½ the width of the bandage.

8. Wrap the bandage firmly and smoothly while holding the roll close to the extremity with the dominant hand.
9. Complete bandaging, with two circular turns and secure with clips or a safety pin.
10. Leave resident in comfortable position in bed or chair.

❧ PROBLEM-SOLVING ACTIONS

1. Allow fingers or toes to be exposed to check circulation when applying elastic bandage.
2. Avoid use of tape to secure ends as this may be difficult to remove with laundering.
3. Avoid unrolling the bandage before application as this would interfere with the even pressure that needs to be achieved to enhance circulation.
4. Elastic bandages should be removed at least every 8 hours or if they become loose or separate at the turns, skin should be washed, dried, checked for integrity when bandage is removed and reapplied.
5. Circulation in the extremity should be assessed every 4 to 8 hours as needed.
6. When more than one roll of the bandage is needed, continue with a second roll with overlapping spiral turns.
7. Bandages may be laundered and rolled for future use.

❧ EVALUATION

Peripheral pulse within baseline parameters, absence of cold, bluish color or pallor to skin or nail beds, absence of edema, numbness, tingling at distal extremity

ANTIEMBOLISM HOSE

Antiembolism hose are elastic stockings (TEDS) applied to an extremity to promote venous return and prevent pooling of blood in the leg(s). They support veins in the leg by compression to prevent deep vein thrombosis. They are indicated for use in those who are experiencing immobility and impaired circulation. They are applied postoperatively to promote circulation. Compression sleeves are available for residents who are experiencing lymphedema following mastectomy to promote lymphatic drainage and reduce edema. Antiembolism hose are available in knee, thigh, and waist lengths. Full length hose provide the firmest stretch below the knee and a reduced stretch above the knee.

ASSESSMENT

Condition of extremities for color and temperature, type of hose to be applied, history of circulatory impairment, reason for application of hose or sleeve

NURSING DIAGNOSES

Altered Tissue Perfusion (Peripheral); Impaired Physical Mobility; High Risk for Impaired Skin Integrity

GOAL

Peripheral circulation within baseline parameters; correct application and monitoring of antiembolism hose or compression sleeve

INTERVENTIONS

Equipment/Supplies

- Antiembolic hose or compression sleeve of correct size and length
- Measuring tape
- Talcum powder
- Warm water, soap, soft towel

Resident

- Explain purpose of procedure and expected results
- Place in position of comfort with extremity exposed

PROCEDURE

1. Perform handwashing.
2. Become familiar with baseline peripheral pulses and skin color and temperature, physician order for length of hose and duration, whether continuous or intermittent.
3. Measure the circumference of the widest part of the calf and from the bottom of heel to the back of the knee if a below-the-knee stocking is to be applied; the circumference of the widest part of the calf and from the bottom of the heel to the gluteal fold if a thigh or full-length stocking is to be applied, and bottom of heel to the waist if a waist-length stocking is to be applied.
4. Wash appropriate limb(s) and pat dry; apply a light layer of talcum powder to facilitate application.

5. Insert dominant hand inside the hose and grasp the heel portion, pull the heel up and turn the hose inside out while leaving the foot apart inside the stocking.

6. Place the foot inside the stocking and ease the toes and foot into it so that the heel is in the correct position for placing into stocking.

7. Complete application of the stocking over the foot by gathering the portion of the hose over the toes and easing this over the heel and up to the ankle.

8. Check that the hose on the foot is smooth and positioned correctly.

9. Grasp the gathered stocking at the ankle with the fingers and ease it up the leg two inches at a time to allow for smoothing of the hose until it is properly placed, depending on the length of hose being applied.

10. Check hose for proper placement of circular opening under the foot, knee and femoral area; and that top of hose is not cuffed.

11. If a second limb is to have hose applied, repeat the procedure.

12. To remove hose, insert fingers inside the top and grasp with hands, pull hose down inside out with firm, smooth movement.

13. Leave resident in comfortable position with no complaints of excessive tightness or wrinkling of hose.

❧ PROBLEM-SOLVING ACTIONS

1. Hose that do not fit properly, are too short, long, or tight cause excessive pressure and compromise circulation.

2. Hose are best applied in the morning when the least amount of blood is present in the veins of the leg.

3. Massaging the legs should be avoided as this may dislodge a thrombus from a vein.

4. Hose should be removed at least every 12 hours and distal circulation assessed at least every 4 hours.

5. Hose should be free of wrinkles or curling at the top.

6. Application of the hose may be performed without talcum if skin is dry; hose should be hand laundered before use if resident has skin sensitivities.

7. Hose may be worn continuously or only when in bed and should be removed and/or applied accordingly.

8. Custom-made hose may be needed if the resident cannot be fitted with standard sizes or if legs are deformed.

9. Hose may be hand laundered with mild soap and warm water, dried and reapplied; a second pair should be available for use while laundering is done.

❧ EVALUATION

Absence of cold, bluish color or pallor to toes or nail beds, absence of numbness, tingling, pain or edema in limb, hose smooth and straight on extremity and aligned correctly

HOLTER MONITOR

The Holter monitor is an electrocardiographic (ECG) device worn by a resident to provide continuous information about the heart action during usual daily activities. The heart action is recorded on tape for 24 to 36 hours which is then scanned using computer technology to detect the presence of arrhythmias. It may also be used to monitor the effects of medication or to evaluate the effects of a pacemaker. When the resident experiences symptoms, an ECG can be utilized for longer periods of time to determine the cause.

ASSESSMENT

Presence of arrhythmias, chest pain, palpitations, history of myocardial infarct or other cardiac conditions, permanent pacemaker insertion, length of time for monitor use and whether continuous or intermittent

NURSING DIAGNOSES

Decreased Cardiac Output; Pain; High Risk for Impaired Skin Integrity

GOALS

Recording of heart activity by device; written recording of activities and responses in a diary

INTERVENTIONS

Equipment/Supplies

- Device properly loaded with a tape
- Electrodes properly attached to chest and recording device
- Battery
- Belt clip or shoulder strap
- Notebook and pencil

Resident

- Explain purpose of procedure and expected results

PROCEDURE

1. Perform handwashing.
2. Check all connections, including those from the electrodes and extension cable and the recorder.
3. Insert a fresh battery into the recorder.
4. Connect the recorder to the waist or shoulder.
5. Tape lead wires together to reduce movement if necessary.
6. Note time and duration that recorder is on.
7. Inform resident to record events in a notebook including the time and symptoms experienced.
8. Conceal recorder under clothing if requested.
9. Reapply any electrode that becomes disconnected or loose.
10. Allow the resident to engage in normal activities.
11. Transport the resident to the agency which will scan the tape and inform the physician of the results.

❧ PROBLEM-SOLVING ACTIONS

1. Avoid allowing the device to get wet or accidently dropped.

2. Have telephone number on hand to call agency that is managing the monitor if needed.

3. Have recorder removed at the conclusion of the procedure.

4. Activity should be encouraged and modified to resemble usual daily activities as much as possible, if there are no restrictions, to detect those arrhythmias caused by any activity.

5. Coordinate therapeutic regimen (dietary, OT, PT, medications) with cardiac monitoring.

6. A small, hand-held ECG unit with a single lead is now also being used that records activity and can be transmitted via telephone for analysis.

❧ EVALUATION

Correct monitoring and identification of heart activities (normal and abnormal)

PERMANENT PACEMAKER

A permanent pacemaker is a device (generator) implanted and sutured into a subcutaneous pocket on the right shoulder with leads attached to the right side of the heart. It is inserted to overcome conduction problems and regulate heart rate.

ASSESSMENT

Type of pacemaker and reason for use, presence of symptoms before pacemaker insertion, history of cardiac condition, presence of pacemaker malfunction, pulses and characteristics

NURSING DIAGNOSES

Decreased Cardiac Output; Altered Tissue Perfusion; High Risk for Injury

GOALS

Correct functioning of pacemaker; circulatory status within baseline parameters; proper monitoring of pacemaker function

INTERVENTIONS

Equipment/Supplies

- Watch with second hand
- Transmitter and electrodes for telephone checks
- Telephone

Resident

- Explain purpose of procedure and expected results

PROCEDURE

1. Perform handwashing.
2. Become familiar with past electrographic readings, baseline parameters for pulses, frequency of pulse and telephone transmitter checks.
3. Check pulse daily for acceptable variations and possible need for generator change.
4. Ground all electrical equipment in the environment and avoid exposure to electromagnetic interferences.
5. Perform a telephone check as follows:
   a. Place electrodes on skin (wrists) when pacemaker clinic requests such placement.
   b. Turn the transmitter on.
   c. Place the telephone on the transmitter with the mouthpiece at the audio output port.
   d. Allow time for the ECG to be transmitted.
   e. Place a magnet over the transmitter if the pacemaker clinic requests this to detect any pacemaker malfunction.
   f. Remove electrodes, cleanse skin, and remove transmitter for storage until the next evaluation.

❧ PROBLEM-SOLVING ACTIONS

1. Use alternate methods of monitoring pacemaker function (magnet over generator before taking pulse) or rate of pacemaker stimulation (use of transistor radio and magnet while taking pulse).

2. Note if demand or pre-set pacemaker present and assess pulse accordingly; a pre-set pacemaker maintains the heart rate and same pulse at all times. A demand pacemaker allows for variations in heart rate and pulse depending on individual needs.

3. Depending on life of generator, prepare for replacement in the future.

4. Suggest loose clothing to be worn over pacemaker generator site.

5. Prepare for cardiopulmonary resuscitation (CPR) if needed and emergency 911 assistance.

6. Review manufacturer's pacemaker instruction guide for information regarding the specific pacemaker and care.

❧ EVALUATION

Absence of dizziness, dyspnea, edema of extremities, telephone evaluation reveals proper pacemaker function with no loss of sensing or loss of capture

RIGHT ATRIAL CATHETER MANAGEMENT

*T*he right atrial catheter is an intravenous line inserted near to or into the right atrium to provide long or short-term central venous access for the administration of fluids, total parenteral nutrition, medications such as chemotherapeutic agents, antibiotics, and to allow for the withdrawal of blood samples to prevent repeated venipunctures. The catheter (Groshong or Hickman) can be inserted via an incision usually in the right upper chest through a subcutaneous tunnel into the cephalic vein and then the superior vena cava for long-term therapy. Another catheter (subclavian) can be inserted via an incision in the neck through the jugular or subclavian vein into the superior vena cava for short-term therapy. The Hickman catheter can include a single or double lumen to allow for continuous and intermittent infusion, and the Groshong catheter has a single or double lumen with a pressure tip that prevents blood from backing up into the catheter between intermittent infusions. This eliminates the need for heparinization.*

Right atrial catheter care includes dressing change (usually every 3 days unless wet, soiled, or loose), cap change (usually if contaminated, following blood withdrawal, or every 3 days), catheter irrigation or heparinization (depending on type of catheter usually before and sometimes following a treatment), catheter removal (when treatments via the catheter are discontinued), withdrawal of blood samples, emergency procedures, and administration of fluids and medications (type and frequency ordered on an individual basis).

ASSESSMENT

Type of catheter and treatments, catheter placement and patency, condition of skin at site and healing around cuff, type of dressing and need for change

NURSING DIAGNOSES

Anxiety; High Risk for Infection; Ineffective Individual Coping; High Risk for Impaired Skin Integrity

GOALS

Right atrial catheter position and patency maintained without complications; correct monitoring and care of catheter

INTERVENTIONS

Equipment/Supplies

- Right atrial catheter of correct size with correct parts and attachments in place
- Infusion pump for continuous infusion
- Sterile dressing tray or individually wrapped sterile packages of dressings, Betadine, alcohol swabs, forceps, clamps, scissors, gloves, face mask
- Sterile injection cap
- Sterile syringes (5 ml), needles (#20, #25)

- Heparin in vial or Tubex unit dose
- Tape, Op-Site or other tape
- Sterile normal saline

- Blood collection tubes and syringe (10 ml)
- Culture tube and necessary container/packaging

<u>Resident</u>

- Explain purpose of procedure and expected results
- Place in position of comfort, low- or semi-Fowler's, sitting position if appropriate

❧ PROCEDURE

1. Perform handwashing.

2. Become familiar with catheter, reason for placement and treatments ordered.

3. Expose catheter site and tract and drape as needed for privacy.

4. If dressing change is needed:
   a. Put on mask and set up sterile field, open packages and gloves near working area on a clean, flat surface.
   b. Gently loosen transparent tape and old dressing with a gloved hand without creating tension on the catheter or touching exit site; dispose in special container.
   c. Put on sterile gloves and cleanse the site with Betadine swabs in circular movements around and away from the catheter using one swab per movement until area 2 inches around the catheter is cleansed; hold catheter away from the skin with the nondominant gloved hand.
   d. After the Betadine dries, cleanse with alcohol swabs in the same manner and allow to dry.
   e. Apply an antiseptic ointment around the catheter exit site and place a small sterile dressing over the site.
   f. Coil the catheter on the small dressing and cover with transparent tape dressing and tape around the edges to form a picture frame appearance.
   g. Tape the catheter to the chest with the cap in an upward direction if more secure attachment is needed or if catheter is not coiled under the dressing.
   h. Remove gloves and discard all used articles appropriate to Universal Precautions.

5. If cap change is needed:
   a. Put on mask and place opened sterile package containing the cap nearby on a clean, flat surface.
   b. Expose the tip of the catheter at the cap site and clamp catheter about 2 inches from the cap area, unless a Groshong is in place (not clamped because of special valve); use special forcep or protect catheter with tape applied at the site of clamping.
   c. Put on sterile gloves, hold catheter while cleansing cap junction with alcohol and Betadine; allow to dry.
   d. Unscrew cap from the catheter while holding the catheter, heparinize the catheter, remove the cover from the new cap and screw or twist cap into place on the catheter, heparinize the catheter again (Groshong does not need heparinization but is irrigated with normal saline following cap change)
   e. Unclamp catheter and retape to chest.
   f. Discard used articles as in other right atrial catheter procedures.

6. If heparinization is needed:
   a. Prepare syringe with appropriate amount (varies with physician) of heparin from a vial or prepared unit dose vial in a Tubex and place nearby on a clean, flat surface; allow medication to warm to room temperature.
   b. Expose cap and cleanse according to procedure.
   c. Insert needle of heparin syringe into the cap and slowly inject the heparin.
   d. Clamp tube 2 inches above the cap site after the last of the heparin is administered.
   e. Remove needle from cap, unclamp the catheter, and retape to the chest.
   f. Discard used articles as in other right atrial catheter procedures.

7. If catheter irrigation is needed:
   a. Prepare a syringe with the correct amount of sterile normal saline.
   b. Expose the cap and cleanse according to the procedure.
   c. Insert needle of syringe into the cap and carefully inject the saline.
   d. Remove the needle while maintaining positive pressure on the plunger during withdrawal.
   e. Discard used articles as for any right atrial catheter procedures.

8. If withdrawal of blood sample is needed:
   a. Prepare heparin or normal saline for specific catheter.
   b. Place labeled blood tubes in an upright position in a glass or holder nearby on a clean, flat surface
   c. Expose and cleanse the cap according to procedure.
   d. Remove the cap and attach a 10 ml syringe to the connector.

    e. Withdraw a small amount of blood (5 ml) and discard with the syringe.

    f. Attach another syringe and withdraw the amount of blood needed for the specimen without applying too much suction.

    g. Place blood in tube, continue withdrawing blood until all specimens are obtained in appropriate tubes.

    h. Place stoppers in tubes and gently shake those as needed after the tubes are filled.

    i. Inject heparin into the cap or saline into the connection after blood is withdrawn depending on type of catheter (Groshong requires 20 ml saline prior to and 10 ml after blood withdrawal).

    j. Attach a new injection cap according to procedure.

    k. Discard used articles as for other right atrial catheter procedures.

    l. Transmit the tubes with specimens in a biohazard bag to the proper laboratory for testing.

9. If catheter removal is needed:

    a. Clamp catheter.

    b. Put on sterile gloves and gently remove the dressings and tape.

    c. Grasp the catheter and, with smooth, slow, firm movements, withdraw it without the use of any force.

    d. Clip the tip of the catheter with a sterile scissors, place in a sterile container, label, and send to the laboratory for culture and possible infection identification.

    e. Apply pressure to the site for 5 minutes with a sterile dressing to control any bleeding

    f. Cleanse site and apply Betadine ointment and dry dressing.

    g. Inspect the catheter for roundness, and smoothness and wholeness and notify the physician if the tip is ragged; that this could indicate that a piece has broken off.

    h. Discard the catheter and articles used as in other right atrial catheter procedures.

10. If emergency or special care is needed:

    a. Clearing a clot from a catheter can be attempted by withdrawing it from the catheter with a syringe until blood is seen in the syringe.

    b. Leaks or breaks in catheter should be covered with sterile dressing, catheter clamped, physician notified.

    c. Some leaks or breaks can be repaired by those with special training for this procedure if the damage is at least 2 inches from the chest wall; this is done by removing the damaged part and replacing it with a new piece of tubing taped in place with a splicing sleeve.

    d. Tube dislodgement should be covered with sterile dressings at the insertion site, clamped, and the physician notified immediately for removal and/or replacement.

11. If intravenous fluid or medication administration is needed:

    a. If intermittent, bolus medications are ordered, prepare the correct dose in a syringe with a needle attached, follow procedure for heparinization or irrigation, inject the medication slowly, heparinize or irrigate according to type of catheter following medication.

    b. If continuous infusion of fluids or medications is ordered, prepare the correct container of fluids with or without medications and connect tubing set-up, expel air, connect to infusion pump set at the correct rate for amount and time, prepare cap according to procedure and connect the intravenous adaptor to the cap; medications via measured container or piggyback intravenous are administered in the same fashion following proper preparation and measurement (see Measured Container, Piggyback Intravenous, Infusion Control Device).

✖ PROBLEM-SOLVING ACTIONS

1. Note catheter damage, cap disconnection, and kinking of catheter when giving care.

2. Protect site from contamination, irritation, or trauma; pulling or tension that can dislodge catheter.

3. Maintain sterility of all articles that come in contact with the catheter at the insertion site.

4. Some catheters have a hub instead of a cap attached at the end and the hub can be removed and replaced in the same manner as the injection cap.

✖ EVALUATION

Absence of redness, pain, swelling at insertion site, catheter patency maintained by heparinization or irrigation, dressing and cap clean and intact, appropriate response to treatments and medications

UNIT IX

PULMONARY PROCEDURES

- Airway Suctioning

- Breathing Exercises, Cough/Deep/Pursed Lip

- Breathing Therapy Devices

- Laryngectomy Stoma Management

- Oxygen Administration

- Postural Drainage

- Tracheostomy Management

AIRWAY SUCTIONING

Suctioning is performed to ensure a patent airway by removing secretions from the nose, pharynx, and trachea. Accumulations of these secretions affect breathing patterns. Suctioning is prescribed for residents unable to clear the airway by coughing due to neuromuscular, neurologic, or pulmonary conditions, debilitating states, unconscious states, or in the presence of an artificial airway (see Tracheostomy Management). The secretions are removed via a catheter inserted into the airway and connected to a suction apparatus. The upper or lower airway or both can be suctioned, depending on individual needs. The upper airway includes the nose, pharynx, and the mouth, and suctioning these areas is referred to as oropharyngeal or nasopharyngeal suctioning. Suctioning is used routinely to remove secretions from the mouth and pharynx to prevent aspiration when swallowing is ineffective. The lower airway includes the trachea and bronchi and is used to remove secretions in those who are unable to cough. This suctioning is performed according to policy by qualified nurses. A sputum specimen can be collected during this procedure.

Clean technique is utilized to perform routine suctioning; sterile technique to perform deep suctioning. The technique is important because of the risk for infection in those with compromised pulmonary function. Suctioning should also be done correctly to prevent irritation or trauma to the mucosa. Other complications to which the nurse should be alert include bradycardia and hypotension from stimulation of the vagus nerve.

❧ ASSESSMENT

Respiration status, airway patency, ability to mobilize and cough up secretions, tachypnea, dyspnea, breath sounds, condition of oral and nasal mucous membranes, frequency of suctioning needed

❧ NURSING DIAGNOSES

Ineffective Airway Clearance; Ineffective Breathing Pattern; High Risk for Infection; High Risk for Aspiration; High Risk for Impaired Tissue Integrity

❧ GOAL

Respiratory rate, depth, and ease maintained with airway patency

❧ INTERVENTIONS

Equipment/Supplies

- Portable or wall suction apparatus
- Oxygen source
- Tubing and connectors
- Correct sized catheter with proper tip
- Disposable unsterile or sterile gloves
- Water soluble lubricant
- Basin with tap water or sterile water or saline
- Tissues, hand towel
- Specimen collection container

Resident

- Explain purpose of procedure and expected results
- Place in low to semi-Fowler's position

❧ PROCEDURE

1. Perform handwashing.

2. Become familiar with the type of suctioning to be performed and the reason and frequency/length of the suctioning.

3. Assemble the suctioning materials with clean container, tubing, and the kit or individually-wrapped supplies for the procedure, pour water in the basin.

4. Place a towel or protective cover over the chest.

5. Perform and maintain medical asepsis for oronasopharyngeal suctioning:
   a. Put on clean, unsterile gloves. Administer oxygen, if ordered.
   b. Measure the catheter from the tip of the nose to the earlobe for length to be inserted.
   c. With the catheter in the dominant hand, connect it to the tubing held in the nondominant hand and turn on the suctioning machine with the nondominant hand and set at 120-150 mm Hg.
   d. Run water through the tubing and test the thumb control, apply water-soluble lubricant to the tip of the catheter.
   e. Insert the measured length of the catheter into the nares toward the pharynx with the thumb off the control while the neck is slightly hyperextended and the mouth open.
   f. Suction for 5 seconds with the thumb on the control and then as the catheter is gently withdrawn, rotate with the thumb on and off the control.
   g. Flush the catheter in the basin of water and allow for a rest period before another thrust is performed.
   h. Reinsert the catheter in the other nares and repeat the suctioning and continue alternating the nares for a period of not longer than 15-30 seconds for the entire procedure.
   i. Suction the mouth at the conclusion of the nasopharyngeal procedure.
   j. If the oral route is used for insertion of the catheter instead of the nares, insert along the side of the oral cavity with the thumb off the control until the oropharynx is reached and proceed to use the control and withdraw the catheter as previously described.

6. Perform and maintain sterile technique for nasotracheal suctioning:
   a. Open the sterile kit or individual packages to access the articles needed.
   b. Oxygenate the resident to prevent hypoxemia during the procedure.
   c. Put on the sterile gloves.
   d. Measure the catheter from the tip of the nose to the earlobe and downward to the thyroid cartilage on the neck.
   e. While holding the catheter with the dominant hand, connect to the tubing held in the nondominant hand and place the catheter in the basin of sterile water; place the thumb on control to allow water to run through and moisten the tip.
   f. Insert the catheter into the nares and, with the head slightly hyperextended, advance it the measured length into the trachea.
   g. Allow coughing to bring up secretions and start to suction while gently rotating the catheter during withdrawal with the thumb on and off the control.
   h. Remove and flush the tubing by placing it in the basin of sterile water with the thumb on the control.
   i. Repeat the procedure and suction each time not to exceed 3-5 minutes for no longer than 15 minutes to complete the procedure.
   j. Allow to rest and oxygenate between each suctioning thrust.
   k. Complete the procedure by suctioning the oral cavity.

7. Dispose of used articles using Universal Precautions; cleanse, disinfect and store reusable supplies and articles.

❧ PROBLEM-SOLVING ACTIONS

1. Suctioning supplies should be at bedside ready for immediate use.

2. Advise resident to continue breathing during the procedure; administer oxygen to avoid further depletion.

3. Inform the resident that one of the purposes of the procedure is to stimulate coughing; allow him to cough.

4. If bronchospasm or laryngospasm occur, cease suctioning and remove catheter.

5. Sterile saline or water can be instilled (3-5 ml) to liquify thick secretions.

6. Avoid using suctioning during insertion of the catheter as this causes trauma to the mucosa.

7. A tongue blade and flashlight can facilitate catheter insertion via the nasal route.

8. Encourage coughing to bring up secretions during the procedure to minimize the number of thrusts needed to clear the airways.

9. Provide oxygen therapy prior to, during, and after the procedure as tracheal suctioning reduces arterial oxygen pressure by 35 mm Hg; this hypoxia can lead to tachycardia, arrhythmias, and cardiac arrest.

≈ EVALUATION

Airway patency maintained with correct and effective suctioning done at appropriate intervals using appropriate technique; no evidence of mucous membrane impairment or hypoxemia

BREATHING EXERCISES, COUGH/DEEP/PURSED LIP

Breathing exercises are performed to improve respiratory function and lung volume by strengthening respiratory muscles removing secretions from the respiratory tract. These exercises include coughing and deep, or diaphragmatic breathing, and pursed-lip breathing to prevent or restore respiratory function in acute or chronic pulmonary diseases. The selection of exercises depends on the reason, such as coughing and deep breathing for preventive and diaphragmatic and pursed-lip breathing for restorative. They can be done with other pulmonary physiotherapy such as postural drainage techniques, incentive spirometry, and intermittent positive pressure breathing (IPPB). Ineffective coughing and ventilation can lead to decreased gas exchange, causing hypoxia, and accumulation of secretions, and lung complications such as pneumonia and atelectasis.

❧ ASSESSMENT

Respirations and characteristics, breath sounds, use of accessory muscles, pulmonary and neuromuscular conditions affecting breathing, medication regimen, exertional dyspnea

❧ NURSING DIAGNOSES

Ineffective Airway Clearance; Ineffective Breathing Pattern; Activity Intolerance; Ineffective Individual Coping; High Risk for Infection

❧ GOAL

Maintenance of optimal respiratory function with patent airway

❧ INTERVENTIONS

Equipment/Supplies

- Pillow
- Mouthwash solution
- Tissues

Resident

- Explain purpose of procedure and expected results
- Place in low-Fowler's or sitting position

❧ PROCEDURE

1. Perform handwashing.
2. Become familiar with the exercises to be performed and the required frequency of each exercise.
3. Perform coughing and deep breathing exercises:
   a. Offer a pillow to place over the abdomen to act as a splint and position in a sitting posture with knees slightly flexed.
   b. Provide tissue during the procedure.
   c. Request to cough once or twice to clear airway.
   d. Request to place hand on lower chest and take a deep breath and note that the hand is elevated.
   e. Request to hold the breath for about 3 seconds and slowly exhale to perform deep breathing; repeat 5-10 times as tolerated.

    f.   To include coughing with the deep breathing procedure, request to take 2 soft breaths followed by a deep breath with the mouth slightly open, hold the breath and cough twice during expiration into the tissue, rest and repeat the coughing procedure 5-10 times as tolerated with a rest between each coughing procedure.

4. Perform pursed-lip breathing exercises:
    a.   Place in semi-Fowler's with the knees slightly flexed as for abdominal breathing exercises.
    b.   Request to take a deep breath through the nose with the mouth closed and to exhale slowly through the mouth with the lips shaped in a whistling position while the abdominal muscles are contracted and breathe out allowing twice the amount of time as for inhaling or until the lungs are as emptied of air as possible.
    c.   Repeat this breathing technique as needed.

5. Perform diaphragmatic breathing exercises:
    a.   Place in same position as for abdominal breathing.
    b.   Request to place one hand on the abdomen and the other hand on the chest and inhale through the nose slowly.
    c.   As the abdomen is felt moving outward during inspiration, request to exhale using pursed-lip breathing as the abdominal muscles are contracted inward.
    d.   Perform 3-4 times with a rest allowed between each exercise.

❧ PROBLEM-SOLVING ACTIONS

1. Positions to perform the exercises can vary from lying, sitting or standing to prepare for effective breathing during different activities.

2. Exercises can be performed from 2-4 times a day (coughing more frequently) depending on fatigue and secretion removal with increases in number of times up to 10 if tolerated.

3. Sputum specimens can be collected during the coughing procedure.

4. Mouthwash can be provided following the coughing procedure.

❧ EVALUATION

Patent airways with effective breathing exercises to remove secretions and maintain respiratory function

BREATHING THERAPY DEVICES

Breathing therapy devices are used to provide inhalation treatments that encourage and sustain inspirations (incentive spirometer), or deliver moisture or medication to the airways and environment (nebulizers, intermittent positive pressure breathing (IPPB) and humidifiers). The effect of these treatments is to decrease the work of breathing, increase lung volume by inflating the lungs, and mobilize and raise secretions. The incentive spirometer is a plastic tube that holds a light-weight ball that moves up with a deep breath and can be measured to determine adequate respiratory flow. Nebulizers are large volume devices to deliver cool or warm mist for long-term therapy or small volume devices to deliver medications (see Medications, Inhalation, Small Volume Nebulizer) or short-term, intermittent treatments that assist in removing secretions. Small volume nebulizers can be held in the hand or attached to a ventilator or IPPB machine. Humidifiers provide moisture to the environment to facilitate breathing. Humidified oxygen prevents drying and irritation to respiratory mucosa. The devices can deliver humidity to the environment and release a cool mist or steam vapor (room humidifier), deliver humidity at the body temperature (cascade humidifier), deliver humidity to mix with a dry gas such as oxygen (cold bubble). IPPB, a device that is not used frequently since the same results can be achieved by the other pulmonary physiotherapy procedures, can deliver medication, oxygen, or environmental air into the lungs by the use of pressure higher than the pressure in the lungs.

❧ ASSESSMENT

Respiratory status, breath sounds, ability to cough up secretions and characteristics of sputum, frequency of treatments, medications to be administered by inhalation, type of device used for treatments

❧ NURSING DIAGNOSES

Ineffective Breathing Pattern; Ineffective Airway Clearance, High Risk for Impaired Tissue Integrity; High Risk for Infection

❧ GOAL

Correct and effective use of breathing device with optimal respiratory function maintained

❧ INTERVENTIONS

Equipment/Supplies

- IPPB machine and proper parts
- Incentive spirometer (flow or volume)
- Humidifier, proper type and connections
- Nebulizer with proper container and connections (large or small volume)
- Tap or sterile distilled water
- Oxygen and/or medications
- Stethoscope
- Tissues

Resident

- Explain purpose of procedure and expected results
- Place in position of comfort

‍‍❧ PROCEDURE

1. Perform handwashing.

2. Become familiar with the therapy to be performed, type of device used, and frequency of treatments.

3. Perform incentive spirometry:
   a. Place in a position that allows for the device to be used in the upright position, sitting or semi-Fowler's.
   b. Connect the tubing and mouthpiece to the device and set the rate for the flow or volume.
   c. Request to exhale slowly and completely and then place the lips over the mouthpiece and inhale, hold the breath until the set level is reached, or as long as possible.
   d. Request to remove the device from the mouth and exhale, encourage to cough.
   e. Request to take 4-5 breaths and repeat the procedure for number of times/hour and frequency during the day depending on reason for use.
   f. Monitor breath sounds prior to and following the procedure and compare changes in air movement in the lungs.

4. Perform IPPB:
   a. Place in high-Fowler's.
   b. Adjust pressure valve to ordered setting, usually 15 cm H_2O.
   c. Set the oxygen rate or prepare and connect the medication nebulizer to be administered, if ordered.
   d. Request to exhale slowly and completely.
   e. Request to close lips over the mouthpiece and not to breathe through the nose, or use a nose clip.
   f. Request to inhale deeply through the mouth to deliver the breath by the machine and to hold the breath following the inspiration.
   g. Request to exhale slowly and continue to breathe normally.
   h. Remove the mouthpiece to allow for coughing and rest when needed.
   i. Repeat the procedure for 15-20 minutes, 2-3 times/day as tolerated.
   j. Monitor pulse, blood pressure, and breath sounds prior to, during, and after treatment to detect changes caused by response to medications or a decrease in cardiac output and venous return.

5. Perform humidification:
   a. Prepare the humidifier by adding distilled water to the reservoir to the line and close or reattach it to the device, check water level during the procedure and refill when needed.
   b. If the device has a temperature control, set it at room temperature or body temperature or as ordered.
   c. Place at the proper distance near the head on a bedside table and close the windows and door for a room humidifier, note that a mist is visible and direct towards the resident.
   d. Attach the oxygen delivery equipment to the bubble diffusion humidifier and turn the oxygen gauge to the ordered rate, note the bubbles in the water when the oxygen is turned on and flowing.
   e. Set the temperature on the cascade humidifier connected to a ventilator and place the attached tubing at a distance to prevent any flow toward the resident, drain condensation from the tubing as needed, monitor temperature to maintain body or other ordered temperature of the humidity produced and delivered.

6. Perform nebulization:
   a. Prepare the nebulizer with the sterile distilled water and/or medication in the container and attach the appropriate tubing to the compressor pump, ultrasonic or IPPB machine.
   b. Attach tubing to the gas delivery device for ultrasonic nebulizer, turn on machine and note misting, request to breathe deeply for 10-15 minutes, encourage to cough and rest when needed, monitor pulse and breath sounds prior to, during, and following treatment.
   c. Attach cup of medication to the IPPB machine and note the mist for the side stream nebulizer, place the mouthpiece in the mouth with the lips closed over it, request to breathe slowly and deeply for 10-15 minutes, encourage to cough and rest when needed, monitor pulse and breath sounds prior to, during, and following treatment.

7. To perform treatment with hand-held nebulizer, see Medications, Inhalation (Small Volume Nebulizer).

8. Disinfect, wash, rinse, and air dry all reusable equipment and store in a clean plastic bag for future use; follow guidelines for universal precautions in the care of and disposal of equipment and supplies.

PROBLEM-SOLVING ACTIONS

1. Vary the positions to accommodate comfort as well as effective use of breathing devices.
2. Monitor pulse, blood pressure, and breath sounds prior to the use of any device to note changes caused by medications administered and stop treatment if increases or bronchospasms are noted.
3. Use suctioning to remove secretions if unable to bring up and expectorate in tissues.
4. Limit treatment if fatigued and unable to continue.
5. Administer treatments before meals to prevent nausea from a full stomach compressing against the lungs.
6. Do not remove dentures when using devices that need a mouthpiece.

EVALUATION

Patent airways with improved respiratory function following breathing treatments

LARYNGECTOMY STOMA MANAGEMENT

Laryngectomy stoma management includes a combination of rehabilitation and instructions to promote self care. Stoma care is performed on a healed, permanent stoma following laryngectomy with a focus on the maintenance of the stoma and adaptation to the changes in lifestyle.

ASSESSMENT

Physical and psychological response to the stoma, voice restoration device used, appearance and condition of stoma, ability to care for stoma and understand precautions

NURSING DIAGNOSES

High Risk for Aspiration; Ineffective Breathing Pattern; Body Image Disturbance; High Risk for Impaired Tissue Integrity; Impaired Verbal Communication

GOAL

Modification of lifestyle to achieve optimal functioning of speech and respiratory system

INTERVENTIONS

Equipment/Supplies

- Stoma shield
- Humidifier
- Petroleum jelly
- Mouthwash, soft toothbrush
- Tissues

Resident

- Explain purpose of procedure and expected results
- Place in position of comfort, usually sitting

PROCEDURE

1. Perform handwashing or request to perform handwashing for self care.
2. Become familiar with impending dysfunction and effect self concept, ability to provide care to stoma and oral hygiene, type of care needed and frequency.
3. Note type of speech technique or device/prosthesis used and rehabilitative therapy by speech pathologist.
4. Wash the area around the stoma daily with mild soap and warm water, rinse, and gently pat dry, remove any dried secretions.
5. Apply protective ointment around the stoma to protect from irritation.
6. Apply and secure a stoma guard over the area, such as a metal or plastic or cloth bib to prevent foreign material from entering the stoma.
7. Advise the patient to lean forward and cover stoma with a tissue when coughing or sneezing to catch secretions.
8. Provide mouthcare with a soft toothbrush and dentifrice or mouthwash and brush teeth and tongue to control odor and promote clean, healthy oral cavity.

9. Provide environmental humidification to maintain moist mucous membranes and liquify secretions, such as humidifier, running hot water in the shower.

10. Inform of special precautions to protect the stoma and prevent complications by wearing a stoma shield to protect from water when bathing, avoid swimming and use of shaving cream or makeup near the stoma.

11. Inform that breathing through the nose is no longer possible and the ability to laugh, smell food or smoke, or taste foods can be impaired or absent.

✺ PROBLEM-SOLVING ACTIONS

1. Stoma can be shielded by a scarf, blouse or shirt as well as more obvious types of shields.

2. Identification emergency card in the wallet or purse can be used instead of Medic-Alert jewelry, if desired, and if resident leaves the facility.

✺ EVALUATION

Daily safe stoma care and progressive adaptation to alteration in daily living patterns; respiratory patency maintained and communication status improved

OXYGEN ADMINISTRATION

xygen therapy includes the administration of oxygen (O_2) in liters/minute (L/min) by cannula or face mask to treat hypoxemic conditions caused by pulmonary or cardiac diseases. O_2 therapy is also prescribed to ensure oxygenation of all body organs and systems. The amount of oxygen by percent of concentration or L/min, and the method of administration, is ordered by the physician. The administration, monitoring of responses, and safety precautions associated with it are performed by the nurse. The nasal cannula delivers 22-30% oxygen and is the most common, inexpensive, and easiest device to use. The face mask delivers up to 100% oxygen, depending on the type and reason for use. Common oxygen sources for long-term administration include cylinder (portable or stationary) or wall system near the resident's bed. Both sources require humidification to prevent drying of mucous membranes and thickening of respiratory secretions.

ASSESSMENT

Type of delivery system, source, amount and length of therapy, respiratory status, chronic pulmonary or cardiac conditions, cyanosis of skin or nail beds

NURSING DIAGNOSES

Impaired Gas Exchange; Ineffective Breathing Pattern; High Risk for Impaired Tissue Integrity; High Risk for Infection; High Risk for Injury

GOAL

Safe and optimal oxygenation for organ function

INTERVENTIONS

Equipment/Supplies

- Oxygen source, cylinder or wall system
- Connecting tubing and nasal cannula or face mask
- Portable cart to carry small tank
- Extra cylinder and supplies
- Oxygen flowmeter and gauges
- Water soluble ointment for nasal mucosa

Resident

- Explain purpose of procedure and expected results
- Place in semi of high-Fowler's position in bed, sitting or ambulatory as able

PROCEDURE

1. Perform handwashing.
2. Become familiar with the type of oxygen administration, medical diagnosis and reason for oxygen, intermittent or continuous use of oxygen, amount to be delivered.
3. Assemble the wall system apparatus:
   a. Attach the flowmeter.
   b. Fill the humidifier container to the marked level with distilled water.

    c. Attach the tubing to the flowmeter and delivery device to be used.

    d. Turn on the flow and set the desired rate, note that the water in the humidifier is bubbling and hold hand near the device to feel the flow.

4. Assemble the cylinder:

    a. Attach the pressure flow regulator.

    b. Fill the humidifier container to the marked level with distilled water and attach to the cylinder.

    c. Attach the tubing to the regulator and the delivery device to be used.

    d. Open the regulator and adjust to the desired rate, note that the water in the humidifier bubbles and hold hand next to the device to feel the flow.

    e. If a small cylinder is used, position and secure it in a portable cart.

5. Place nasal cannula, usually used for flow rate under 6L/minute, in the nares with the prongs straight or curving downward and around the ears and under the chin, adjust to a snug fit and pad areas on the face and ears with gauze to protect from pressure of the tubing.

6. Place mask, usually used for flow rate over 6L/minute, over nose and mouth and adjust elastic band for a snug fit, pad areas on face with gauze to protect from pressure.

7. Turn on oxygen after properly setting for volume and place device in position.

8. Change device and tubing when needed and wash cannula, mask, tubing with warm water and mild soap and rinse well, allow to air dry, soak in disinfectant solution for 10 minutes q2-3 days and rinse well, air dry and store in a clean plastic bag for reuse, humidifier can also be washed, rinsed and dried every 24 hours when needed and refilled with water and stored dry when not in use.

9. Place NO SMOKING signs in area when oxygen is administered and store in an area free of inflammable substances; avoid use of electrical appliances in the area such as radios, electric razors, hair dryer.

❧ PROBLEM-SOLVING ACTIONS

1. Remove mask at least every 8 hours and for eating and bathing the face; change tubing and mask every 24-48 hours.

2. Check tanks and change when they drop below 500 pounds pressure, bleed the flow meter when O_2 is concluded to eliminate O_2 in the meter when the tank is turned off.

3. Assess oral and nasopharynx mucous membranes for dryness, face and ears for redness and soreness; apply lubricant to the nares and face and change the position of the protective pads every 4 hours.

4. Assess for untoward effects of oxygen administration such as toxicity, hypoventilation, dehydration.

5. Allow the resident to feel the flow of oxygen through the tubing before placing the device on the face.

❧ EVALUATION

Oxygenation maintained with safe and effective delivery of prescribed amount of oxygen

POSTURAL DRAINAGE

Postural drainage is a combination of vibration and percussion to loosen secretions and positioning to remove secretions by gravity. It is done to clear the airways for optimal air flow and prevent pulmonary infection caused by stasis of secretions. The procedure is most commonly done to improve ventilation in those residents who are immobilized as well as in residents with chronic obstructive diseases and neuromuscular conditions.

❧ ASSESSMENT

Respiratory status, breath sounds, ability to cough up secretions, frequency and length of treatment, respiratory disease, need for oxygen administration, weakness, fatigue

❧ NURSING DIAGNOSES

Ineffective Airway Clearance; Ineffective Breathing Pattern; High Risk for Infection; Activity Intolerance

❧ GOAL

Maintenance of patent airway with removal of secretions

❧ INTERVENTIONS

Equipment/Supplies

- Pillows
- Emesis basin and tissues
- Mouthwash solution

Resident

- Explain purpose of procedure and expected results
- Place in position needed for segmental drainage

❧ PROCEDURE

1. Perform handwashing.
2. Become familiar with techniques to be used, frequency/length of treatment, segments to be drained, time of day for treatment.
3. Administer ordered bronchodilators prior to the procedure.
4. Encourage coughing and deep breathing after each segment drained, coughing after vibration or percussion, suction if needed.
5. Encourage activity and movement after each treatment to promote secretion removal.
6. Provide an emesis basin and tissues to hold during the procedure.
7. Support body with pillows during positioning.
8. Drain apical segments in sitting position and leaning back against or forward over a pillow.
9. Drain anterior segments in supine position with a pillow under the knees and the head tilted downward.
10. Drain lateral segments in sidelying position, left and right with a pillow between the legs and head tilted downward.

11. Drain posterior segments of upper lobes in sidelying position with a pillow between the legs and under the chest, of lower lobes in prone position with a pillow under the chest and the head tilted downward.

12. Drain middle segment in supine position slightly sidelying with a pillow between the legs and the head tilted downward.

13. Perform vibration technique in prone position and vibrating the hands in a downward motion on the back chest wall during exhalation.

14. Perform percussion technique in prone position and cup fingers while using clapping, rhythmic movements created by flexion and extension of the wrists.

15. Perform postural drainage treatment for 5-15 minutes in each position, 2-4 times/day, vibration following postural drainage 4-5 times, percussion for 1-2 minutes following postural drainage, any of which should depend on presence of weakness, fatigue or activity intolerance.

❧ PROBLEM-SOLVING ACTIONS

1. Provide mouthwash and oral care following treatments to clear mouth of secretions.

2. Breath sounds should be assessed prior to and following treatments to determine air flow.

3. Use a tilt table, if available, to achieve the head downward position.

4. Administer supplemental oxygen if needed in conjunction with the therapy.

5. Divide session for therapy based on endurance and tolerance level to the activity and positioning, allow for rest periods periodically during the treatment.

6. Avoid performing vibration and percussion on bare skin over spine, kidneys, breasts to prevent injury.

❧ EVALUATION

Secretions mobilized and removed, airway patency maintained with correct performance of postural drainage procedures

TRACHEOSTOMY MANAGEMENT

Tracheostomy management involves routine care procedures such as dressing change and care of the skin surrounding the tracheostomy, cleansing and changing the tracheostomy tube, tracheal suctioning of secretions via the tracheostomy, and changing the ties that hold the tracheostomy tube in place. This procedure is focused on the management of a tracheostomy during the convalescence period following the surgical procedure. The placement of the tracheostomy is below the first or second cartilage, and the procedure is performed to provide a long or short-term artificial airway. It is performed in those who can eventually resume normal breathing patterns or need a permanent airway following a laryngectomy and eventual stoma formation without the need for tube insertion (see Laryngectomy Stoma Management). The procedures are performed with sterile technique.

❧ ASSESSMENT

Respiratory status, breath sounds, type of tube and whether temporary or permanent tracheostomy, condition of trach site, ability to bring up secretions and characteristics of sputum, need for humidification of oxygen, pain, drainage, edema at site

❧ NURSING DIAGNOSES

Ineffective Airway Clearance; Ineffective Breathing Pattern, Impaired Verbal Communication; High Risk for Infection; High Risk for Impaired Skin Integrity; Body Image Disturbance, Anxiety

❧ GOALS

Safe and effective care of tracheostomy site, airway patency and skin integrity maintained, alternative communication methods adopted

❧ INTERVENTIONS

Equipment/Supplies

- Suction equipment and disposable supplies
- Clean, disposable gloves
- Correct size and type of tube
- Gauze dressings, telfa or protective skin stomahesive dressing
- Twill tapes
- Sterile gloves

- Two basins
- Hydrogen peroxide, normal saline or distilled water
- Small brush or pipe cleaners
- Clamp and syringe
- Ointment for skin protection
- Resuscitation bag

Resident

- Explain purpose of procedure and expected results
- Place a hand towel over the chest

- Place in semi or high-Fowler's position in bed or sitting position

❧ PROCEDURE

1. Perform handwashing.

2. Become familiar with procedures needed and frequency, type of tube in place, condition of skin, characteristics of secretions, equipment and supplies to be maintained at bedside.

3. Perform skin care and dressing change:
   a. Set up a sterile field and place needed supplies on the field (see Wound Care, Dressing Change).
   b. Put on gloves and gently remove soiled dressing without manipulating the tube.
   c. Put on sterile gloves and suction the tube at this time, if needed.
   d. Cleanse the skin around and under the neck plate with sterile saline or distilled water, allow to dry.
   e. Prepare the sterile dressing, cut a slit to fit around the tube, and place around the tube from the top to bottom, use telfa or a skin protector type dressing.
   f. Discard the used articles according to universal precautions.

4. Perform tube change and cleansing:
   a. Assemble and prepare basins of hydrogen peroxide and distilled water and other supplies needed.
   b. Put on gloves.
   c. Steady the neck plate with the nondominant hand, unlock and remove the inner cannula with an upward and outward movement with the dominant hand.
   d. Place the inner tube in the basin of hydrogen peroxide and cleanse with the brush or pipe cleaners, rinse with distilled water.
   e. Suction the outer cannula, if needed.
   f. Reinsert the inner cannula with the curve of the tube pointing downward and lock without manipulating the neck plate or outer cannula.
   g. Dispose of used articles using universal precautions.

5. Perform tie change:
   a. Prepare the two twill tapes by cutting a slit 1 inch from the ends.
   b. Cut the soiled tapes and remove from the tube.
   c. Insert each tie through the slots on the side of the neck plate and insert the other ends of each tie through the slit and pull them through to form a loop.
   d. Tie the ends of the tapes at the sides of the neck using square knots.
   e. Trim the excess ends of the tapes and place the small finger between the tape and neck to check for firmness and stability.

6. Perform tracheal suctioning via the tracheostomy:
   a. Assemble and prepare the appropriate catheter and tubing.
   b. Put on sterile gloves; hyperventilate and instill sterile normal saline solution into tracheostomy.
   c. Lubricate catheter tip with water and run water from a basin through the tubing with the machine on.
   d. Insert the catheter 5 inches into the inner cannula of the tube with the dominant hand and the thumb off the control.
   e. Apply suction intermittently using the thumb control while rotating and withdrawing the catheter; limit each insertion and suctioning to 5 seconds.
   f. Place the catheter in the basin of distilled water to clear.
   g. Allow for a rest period between each suctioning attempt.
   h. Suction the mouth and pharynx following the tracheal suctioning.

7. Perform cuff inflation and deflation:
   a. Assemble and prepare supplies needed to suction, remove and insert air and clamp cuffed tracheostomy tube.
   b. Suction before deflating the cuff.
   c. Remove the clamp and attach a 5-10 ml syringe to the tube and withdraw the air from the cuff, note amount of air removed based on size of the cuff.
   d. Suction the lower airway.
   e. Slowly reinject the same amount of air with the syringe and compare with the amount withdrawn.
   f. Clamp the inflation tube and check tube for leakage by noting air escaping from the nose, mouth, or tracheostomy site.

8. Dispose of used articles according to Universal Precautions, cleanse and disinfect reusable articles and store in a clean plastic bag or cover with a clean towel.

9. Provide method of communication such as pencil and paper, magic slate, or other techniques.

10. Provide environmental humidification as needed (see Breathing Therapy Devices).

❧ PROBLEM-SOLVING ACTIONS

1. Extra tracheostomy tube and other essential supplies should always be available; a resuscitation bag should also be available.

2. Tracheostomy should always be protected from possible foreign substance aspiration that can cause infection.

3. Assess for tube displacement and intervene to correct by replacing the outer cannula using an obturator.

4. Allow for as much self-care as possible in maintaining the tracheostomy, provide a mirror on a stand and assist to set up the supplies.

5. Determine schedule for suctioning and care depending on need to maintain an airway free of secretions and skin free of irritation.

6. Provide mouth care as frequently as needed to promote comfort and prevent dryness and odor.

7. Monitor breath sounds and respiratory status every 4 hours while tracheostomy tube is in place.

❧ EVALUATION

Tracheostomy tube and site care provided every 8 hours or as needed, airway patent, skin intact, wound clean

UNIT X

RENAL/UROLOGIC PROCEDURES

- Catheterization, Female/Male
- Catheterization, Intermittent Urethral/Continent Vesicostomy
- Catheter Management
- Intake and Output
- Peritoneal Dialysis
- Toileting, Bedpan/Urinal
- Toileting, Commode/Bathroom
- Urinary Diversion Mangement
- Urinary Incontinence Management

CATHETERIZATION, FEMALE/MALE

Female and male catheterization is the insertion of a catheter into the urinary bladder via the urethra to drain the bladder of urine. Catheterization can be performed using a straight catheter to drain urine from the bladder and then removing it or by using an indwelling catheter that provides continuous drainage. The single catheterization is done to instill medications, relieve retention caused by an enlarged prostate gland, or to drain residual urine that can cause urinary stasis and bladder infection. An indwelling catheter provides continuous bladder drainage in patients with a neurogenic bladder or urinary dysfunction. The suprapubic site can also be catheterized. This involves the insertion of an indwelling catheter into an incision in the lower abdomen that connects with the bladder. Urinary catheterization is performed only when necessary and is usually reserved for a specific purpose and restricted to short-term treatment. Sterile technique is utilized as the bladder is a sterile cavity, and infection associated with catheterization is common.

ASSESSMENT

Reason for catheterization, size and type of catheter, meatal or suprapubic site for irritation, trauma, pain, characteristics of urinary output, I&O every 8 hours for fluid balance

NURSING DIAGNOSES

High Risk for Infection; High Risk for Injury; Urinary Retention; Body Image Disturbance

GOAL

Safe and correct catheterization procedure

INTERVENTIONS

Equipment/Supplies

- Catheterization kit or individually wrapped sterile drape, gloves, antiseptic and swabs, syringe filled with sterile water, basin, specimen container, lid and label

- Sterile dressings and tape for suprapubic care

- Catheter, straight or Foley of proper size

- Drainage system (bag and tubing)

- Water soluble lubricant

- Disposable bag for used articles

Resident

- Explain purpose of procedure and expected results

- Place female in recumbent and male in supine positions and drape for privacy

PROCEDURE

1. Perform handwashing.

2. Become familiar with reason for catheter insertion, site of catheterization, type and size of catheter, need for I&O monitoring and/or specimen collection.

3. Assemble articles on a sterile field including gloves, or open the sterile catheterization kit containing the articles in order of use.

4. Place protective pad under the buttocks to protect the linens.
5. Perform female urethral catheterization:
   a. Put on sterile gloves.
   b. Place the sterile drape under the buttocks.
   c. Place the sterile fenestrated drape over the genitalia.
   d. Separate the labia with the thumb and forefinger of the nondominant hand and cleanse the area from far sides inward with strokes from front to back using a new swab for each stroke and cleansing the meatus last, if cotton balls and antiseptic are used, pick up and cleanse with a forcep to avoid contaminating the sterile, gloved hand.
   e. Pick up the lubricated catheter about one inch from the tip and place the end in the basin to collect the urine with the dominant hand while still holding the labia apart with the nondominant hand.
   f. Insert the catheter about two inches into the meatus or until urine flows into the basin.
   g. Pinch the catheter and urine to flow into the specimen container if needed, cover and place to the side for future labeling.
   h. Allow the bladder to empty of urine and gently withdraw if a single catheterization is being performed.
   i. If an indwelling catheter has been inserted, attach a syringe filled with the proper amount of distilled water to match the capacity of the bag and inject to test the balloon, and then remove after insertion, inject the same amount into the port that leads to the balloon to be inflated.
   j. Gently tug on the catheter to ensure a proper and secure placement in the urinary bladder, connect the catheter end to a closed drainage system; tape the catheter over the leg and to the thigh or use a catheter strap.
   k. Remove gloves and used articles and dispose according to Universal Precautions.
   l. Place in position of comfort.
6. Perform male urethral catheterization:
   a. Put on gloves.
   b. Place the sterile drape over the legs below the penis.
   c. Hold the penis and retract the foreskin (if present) with the nondominant hand and cleanse from the meatus outward in a circular motion with antiseptic swabs or cotton balls with an antiseptic held with a forcep.
   d. Pick up the catheter four inches from the tip, place the end in the basin to collect the urine, and, while holding the penis forward and upward with the nondominant hand, insert the lubricated catheter about seven inches; avoid using any force during the insertion if resistance is met.
   e. Pinch catheter and collect a specimen if needed and then allow the urine to continue to flow into the basin until the bladder is empty if a single catheterization is being performed.
   f. If an indwelling catheter is being inserted, test it with the injection of the proper amount of distilled water into the balloon inflation port before insertion into the meatus, withdraw the fluid and proceed to insert the catheter as above, but with an additional ¾ inch inserted to prevent pressure at the neck of the bladder.
   g. Reinflate the balloon when the catheter is in place through the port with a syringe filled with the proper amount of distilled water for balloon capacity.
   h. Gently tug on the catheter to ensure secure placement, attach the end to a closed drainage system.
   i. Remove gloves and dispose with other used articles according to Universal Precautions.
   j. Tape the catheter to the upper thigh portion of the leg or use a catheter strap.
   k. Place in position of comfort.
7. Perform suprapubic catheterization:
   a. Put on sterile gloves and remove any dressings at the site, discard in bag.
   b. Place the sterile fenestrated drape over the site.
   c. Cleanse around the site with antiseptic swabs from inside outward in a circular motion.
   d. Check the balloon bag on the catheter as outlined above, lubricate the catheter and, holding 4 inches from the tip, insert into the opening to the bladder.
   e. Inject the distilled water into the balloon port of the catheter, remove the syringe and gently tug on the catheter to ensure that it is anchored.
   f. Attach the end of the catheter to a closed drainage system and tape the catheter to the abdomen.
   g. Reapply a sterile gauze dressing at the site, administer ointment to the skin around the site if ordered.
   h. Remove gloves and discard with other used articles according to Universal Precautions.

8. Perform removal of indwelling catheter:
    a. Remove tape from thigh.
    b. Put on disposable gloves.
    c. Attach empty syringe to the balloon port and withdraw the amount of solution that is equal to the amount instilled.
    d. Disconnect the catheter from the drainage system and clamp or pinch closed.
    e. Gently withdraw the catheter and inspect for intactness.
    f. Cleanse the area and pat dry.
    g. Discard the catheter with other used articles according to universal precautions.
    h. Place in position of comfort.

⮞ PROBLEM-SOLVING ACTIONS

1. Assessment of insertion site and urine patterns should be performed prior to this procedure.

2. Fluid intake should be increased to accommodate urinary flow if an indwelling catheter is inserted.

3. Any contamination of the catheter during the procedure requires that a new catheter and/or other sterile articles be used.

4. A sidelying position can be used for female catheterization if weakness or other medical condition makes it difficult to assume the recumbent position.

5. Failure to obtain a return flow should be reported and the balloon should not be inflated.

⮞ EVALUATION

Safe, straight or indwelling catheter insertion or removal at the meatal or suprapubic site for a female or male performed

CATHETERIZATION, INTERMITTENT URETHRAL/ CONTINENT VESICOSTOMY

*I*ntermittent catheterization is the periodic emptying of the bladder performed by the resident or nurse using a straight catheter. It is done via the urethral route or through a stoma created for entry into a bladder pouch (continent vesicostomy). Urethral intermittent catheterization is performed as an alternative to an indwelling catheter to promote urinary continence and allow independence in the control of voiding. It allows the resident to regulate a urinary bladder emptying schedule. Continent vesicostomy intermittent catheterization is performed to empty a surgically-constructed bladder pouch done to correct neurogenic bladder conditions. This urinary diversion does not require the use of an external appliance to collect the urine; instead, a nipple valve is created that only allows for urine removal with a catheter.

Intermittent catheterizations require clean technique if the resident is responsible for the procedure, a combination of sterile and clean technique if the nurse performs the procedure. Both depend on health status, type and availability of supplies, and condition of the urinary bladder and entry site.

❧ ASSESSMENT

Urinary pattern of elimination and amounts, type of catheterization, ability to perform or assist with the procedures and care of supplies, presence of urinary bladder infection or other urologic disorder

❧ NURSING DIAGNOSES

Anxiety; High Risk for Infection; Self-Care Deficit, Toileting; Altered Elimination Patterns

❧ GOAL

Effective intermittent urinary catheterization with minimal or absence of complications

❧ INTERVENTIONS

Equipment/Supplies

- Straight rubber catheters
- Basin to collect urine
- Cleansing swabs
- Commercial kits for single catheterization procedure

- Disposable gloves

- Mirror on a stand

Resident

- Explain purpose of procedure and expected results

- Place in dorsal recumbent or supine position and drape for privacy

❧ PROCEDURE

1. Perform handwashing.

2. Become familiar with catheterization route, frequency and technique for performing the procedure, ability to perform self-catheterization.

3. Assist and instruct to perform intermittent urethral catheterization:
   a. Have resident wash hands.
   b. Assemble the supplies nearby and prepare for use, wipe and lubricate the catheter.
   c. Have resident stand near toilet with one foot on the floor and one on the toilet or assume recumbent position if female; assume standing position next to the toilet if male.
   d. Situate mirror to view the genitalia if female.
   e. Separate the labia with the nondominant hand and wash from front to back with the wipes if female; retract foreskin, if uncircumcised, and wash tip of penis if male.
   f. Instruct or perform insertion of the catheter two to three inches into the meatus while holding the labia apart if female; insert the catheter six inches into the meatus while holding the penis at a right angle if male.
   g. Allow the urine to flow into a container or toilet until the bladder is empty.
   h. Instruct to or pinch the catheter when the flow ceases and withdraw.
   i. Cleanse the catheter with soap and warm water, air dry, and store in a plastic bag or wrap in a clean towel; boil or disinfect if cleansing after using the catheter twice and store for future use.
   j. If using a sterile kit, maintain sterility of the articles and insert the catheter that is connected to a bag that serves to collect the urine, dispose of the articles according to Universal Precautions when the procedure is completed.

4. Assist and instruct to perform intermittent continent vesicostomy catheterization:
   a. Have resident wash hands.
   b. Assemble the supplies nearby and prepare; clean lubricated catheter, antiseptic wipes, container for the urine, gauze dressing and tape.
   c. Place in supine position, drape and put on gloves.
   d. Remove the gauze dressing cover from the stoma and clean the stoma and peristomal area using a circular motion from the inside outward.
   e. Hold the lubricated catheter in the dominant hand and insert into the stoma with the end resting in a container.
   f. Allow the urine to flow into the container, pinch the catheter when the flow ceases and remove; if the urine does not flow, gently apply suction with a syringe to start the flow.
   g. Dry the peristomal area and apply a gauze bandage over the stoma, tape in place.
   h. Cleanse the used catheter with soap and water, air dry and store in a plastic container or wrap in a towel; disinfect when cleansing and rinse well before drying and storing.

❧ PROBLEM-SOLVING ACTIONS

1. Assessment of stoma condition and peristomal skin for irritation and urine for cloudiness and foul odor indicating bladder infection.

2. Use calibrated container to collect the urine if I&O is being monitored.

3. Assist and encourage to perform self-catheterization at the appropriate times and to adapt to the procedure, provide written instructions if needed.

4. Collect a urine specimen for laboratory examination if needed.

❧ EVALUATION

Daily maintenance of urinary elimination by intermittent catheterization, effective urethral or vesicostomy self-catheterization at appropriate intervals

CATHETER MANAGEMENT

Catheter management is the routine care administered when an indwelling urinary catheter is in place. This routine care protects the resident from infection, injury, and promotes comfort. The procedures include cleansing the genitalia and or the insertion site of the catheter (urethral or suprapubic), dressing change, if appropriate (suprapubic), catheter irrigation or instillation to ensure patency, and care of the closed drainage system.

Both clean and sterile techniques are utilized to perform these procedures; sterile for those that involve the introduction of solution or medication into the urinary bladder (irrigation, instillation) and clean for routine catheter care.

ASSESSMENT

Reason for indwelling catheter, maintenance and patency of catheter, characteristics of urine and presence of cloudiness or foul odor, insertion site for redness, irritation, swelling, pain, cleanliness, bleeding or other drainage

NURSING DIAGNOSES

High Risk for Infection; High Risk for Impaired Tissue Integrity; Body Image Disturbance; Ineffective Individual Coping; High Risk for Injury; Altered Urinary Elimination Patterns

GOAL

Continuous drainage of urine via indwelling catheter with appropriate care and absence of complications

INTERVENTIONS

Equipment/Supplies

- Catheter care kit or antiseptic swabs, gloves, gauze squares, protective drape
- Mild soap, warm water in a basin, towel and washcloth
- Disposable gloves
- Protective pad
- Squeeze bottle with solution

- Drainage bag and tubing or leg bag and straps
- Irrigation solution, syringe and container
- Antibiotic or antiseptic ointment
- Bath blanket

Resident

- Explain purpose of procedure and expected results
- Drape for privacy

- Place in recumbent position for female and supine position for male

PROCEDURE

1. Perform handwashing.
2. Become familiar with procedures to be performed, frequency, need for sterile or clean technique, effect on body image and self-esteem, need for I&O monitoring or specimen collection.

3. Assemble supplies needed for specific care procedures to be performed.

4. Place protective pad under buttocks to protect bed linens.

5. Perform cleansing and care of catheter insertion site:
   a. Put on gloves.
   b. After appropriate positioning, cleanse genitalia by washing from front to back with soap and warm water in female and washing penis in male.
   c. Separate labia with thumb and forefinger of nondominant hand and cleanse the area while holding and applying gentle traction on it; using antiseptic swabs or applicators with antiseptic with downward strokes and around the catheter solution; use a new swab for each stroke and to cleanse the catheter six inches from the insertion site.
   d. Hold the penis with the nondominant hand, retract the foreskin, if needed, cleanse the area with a circular motion and around the catheter using antiseptic swabs, use a new swab for each circle and to cleanse the catheter six inches from the site.
   e. Rinse the area with solution in a squeeze bottle, pat dry with a small towel.
   f. Apply an antiseptic or antibiotic ointment around the catheter at the insertion site.

6. Perform catheter irrigation to relieve obstruction:
   a. Pour sterile irrigation solution into the container.
   b. Untape the catheter from its position and place the sterile drape around the junction of the catheter and tubing to the drainage system.
   c. Cleanse the junction with an antiseptic swab and clamp the catheter.
   d. Disconnect the catheter from the tubing and wrap the tubing end with a sterile gauze square, place in a secure position nearby.
   e. Withdraw 30 ml of solution from the container into the bulb syringe and remove the bulb plunger and insert the tip into the catheter, unclamp the catheter, raise the syringe and allow the solution to flow into the catheter by gravity.
   f. Remove the syringe and allow the fluid to return by gravity into a basin placed between the legs.
   g. Repeat the irrigation twice until the catheter is cleared and urine flows into the basin.
   h. At the conclusion, remove the syringe and reconnect the catheter to the tubing without contaminating the ends, retape the catheter in its appropriate position.
   i. Maintain sterility of irrigation supplies if used frequently, replace with new disposable irrigation kit when needed, dispose of used articles according to Universal Precautions, disinfect and store those articles that are reusable.

7. Maintain closed drainage system:
   a. Secure attachment of tubing to the catheter and note any leakage before taping the catheter in place, allow some slack in the tubing before taping to the leg (some catheters come already attached to the bag).
   b. Keep drainage bag below the level of the bladder to prevent backflow and bladder distention; note kinking in the tubing that can interfere with patency and free flow of urine; never allow bag to be raised above level of the bladder or the bag or tubing to touch the floor.
   c. If catheter is attached to a leg bag, cleanse the catheter tip and tubing end before connecting, position on the thigh or leg and secure the straps below the knee or at the leg.
   d. Empty the bag periodically depending on size or when 2/3 full of urine to prevent pull on the catheter and possible injury caused by weight of a full bag.
   e. Empty the bag by unclamping the drainage tube, allowing the urine to drain into a calibrated container, cleansing the tip after drainage and tucking it back into the pocket to maintain cleanliness and prevent exposure to any contamination.
   f. Change the drainage system with each catheter change according to facility policy or when needed.
   g. Dispose of used articles according to Universal Precautions.

❧ PROBLEM-SOLVING ACTIONS

1. Assessment of insertion site and urine should be performed every 8 hours when an indwelling catheter is in place.

2. Frequency of catheter care is individually determined but should always be performed at least two times/day and after bowel elimination.

3. Avoid manipulation of the catheter during care procedure to prevent injury.

4. Irrigation solution that does not return should be reported.

5. Irrigation can also be done with a syringe and needle through a special port in the catheter and drained via the drainage bag, although this is usually reserved for instillation of medication in which the catheter is clamped for a period of time.

6. Measure all urine because I&O is essential when a patient has a catheter.

7. Fluid intake should be increased to accommodate urinary flow when a catheter is in place.

8. The large drainage bag is preferred; a leg bag can be used but should be discarded and replaced daily.

9. The tips or bags of the drainage system that are contaminated when emptying the bag requires a new sterile drainage bag and tubing set-up be connected to the catheter and the contamination discarded.

10. Suprapubic insertion site can require a dressing around the catheter and a skin barrier to protect the skin from irritation.

❧ EVALUATION

Daily correct and effective management of all aspects of catheter care, absence of urinary bladder infection or tissue injury

INTAKE AND OUTPUT

Intake and output (I&O) is the measurement of fluids taken in or introduced into the body, and fluids eliminated or removed from the body by any route. It is done to calculate and compare the timed or daily totals of each in the evaluation of existing or potential fluid balance problems. Intake includes all fluids and the foods that become liquid at room temperature that are taken orally, all parenteral infusions and injections, and all body instillations or irrigations. Output includes all urine voided, drainage from suction or wound, fluids aspirated from the body, fluids lost in diarrhea, perspiration (sensible loss) and respiration (insensible loss), and blood loss. All fluids are measured with calibrated containers or estimated and amounts recorded on flow sheets for evaluation of totals at 8 to 24-hour intervals. Accuracy in I&O depends on correct measurement, estimation and recording of fluids by the resident and staff members. Fluid intake should average 2500 ml/day unless restricted. I & O that is less than this amount should be closely monitored and evaluated.

ASSESSMENT

History of conditions indicating a need for I&O monitoring, signs and symptoms of fluid imbalance, amount and type of fluid that needs to be measured or estimated other than voiding and drinking, medication regimen that can affect I&O, dietary or fluid restrictions that can affect I&O, serial body weights

NURSING DIAGNOSES

High Risk for Fluid Volume Deficit, Diarrhea, Fluid Volume Excess, Altered Urinary Elimination Pattern

GOAL

Accurate measurement and estimation of I&O

INTERVENTIONS

Equipment/Supplies

- Collection devices, calibrated and non-calibrated (bedpan, urinal, collection containers)
- I&O record and paper/pencil
- Calibrated containers for measurements
- I&O flow sheet

Resident

- Explain purpose for procedure and expected results

PROCEDURE

1. Perform handwashing before and after collection and measurement.

2. Become familiar with types of I&O to be measured and recorded, ability of resident to assist in monitoring and recording fluids.

3. Place an I&O sign on bed and in bathroom to remind of measurement of all fluids to be recorded.

4. Measure and record all liquids ingested, IV fluids, fluids given with medication, enteral fluids, irrigants or instillations not withdrawn or drained.

5. Estimate and record all foods and ice that become liquid at room temperature.

6. Instruct and request resident to record fluids taken between meals on a record placed at the bedside; if resident can't record fluids, measure amount in pitcher at the beginning and end of shift or more frequently if needed.

7. Measure and record all fluids voided from a catheter, vomitus, diarrhea stools, drainage from nasogastric tube, ostomy pouches, fluids aspirated from body cavities.

8. Estimate and record any blood loss, sensible or insensible loss, wound drainage.

9. Inform the resident to void in the urinal or bedpan or collection in the toilet and to avoid discarding the tissue in the urine or voiding in the toilet.

10. Convert the amounts in containers to ml or use calibrated containers in the metric system to record I&O.

11. Record each type of intake and output in the appropriate column on the flow sheet, total and evaluate every 8 hours and compare for fluid balance; record 24 hour totals and compare for positive or negative balance.

❧ PROBLEM-SOLVING ACTIONS

1. Measurement in a calibrated container is preferable to estimating amounts of fluids.

2. Use the agency list to determine the amounts each container holds.

3. Note losses from vomitus or nasogastric drainage and diarrhea that can cause electrolyte imbalances and alkalosis and acidosis respectively.

4. Calculate fluid needs for each individual and use this baseline for determining daily needs, intake should be slightly more than output (positive balance).

5. Monitor daily weight if gains or losses in a specific amount of time are needed to assess fluid excess or deficit when indicated by medical diagnosis (congestive heart failure, chronic renal failure) and/or medication (diuretic) and dietary (low sodium) regimens.

❧ EVALUATION

Proper and accurate I&O measurement every 8 to 24 hours indicating fluid and electrolyte balance.

PERITONEAL DIALYSIS

Peritoneal dialysis is a procedure that involves the removal of waste particles from the blood performed on patients with chronic renal failure. Fluid, electrolytes, toxic substances and waste products are removed using the peritoneum as the dialyzing surface. A dialysate solution is instilled (inflow) into the peritoneal cavity via a peritoneal catheter inserted by the physician and left there for a period of time (dwell). This permits the diffusion (movement from a higher concentration to a lower concentration) of the impurities from the blood to the dialysate solution which is then removed from the peritoneal cavity (outflow). Peritoneal dialysis can be performed manually for continuous ambulatory (CAPD) or for intermittent (IPD) administration. It can also be administered and controlled with an automated cycler machine. Procedures for peritoneal dialysis include preparation and care of the site and catheter, preparation of the dialysate, setting up and performing the inflow and outflow of the dialysate, securing the empty solution pouch around the waist with a belt in CAPD. The most common complications of the procedure are peritonitis from failure in aseptic technique, respiratory distress from the pressure against the diaphragm during inflow, protein depletion as the protein is diffused into the dialysate, hypovolemia from excessive fluid loss, and hypertension, or pulmonary edema from excessive fluid retention.

All procedures for peritoneal dialysis are performed utilizing strict sterile technique.

ASSESSMENT

Type of dialysis (IPD or CAPD), amount and type of dialysate, weight, T, P, BP, before and after dialysis, catheter site for irritation, edema, pain, drainage, characteristics of dialysate return, I&O balance every 8 hours

NURSING DIAGNOSES

High Risk for Infection; High Risk for Impaired Skin Integrity; Anxiety; Fluid Volume Excess; Pain; Powerlessness; Ineffective Individual Coping

GOALS

Safe and effective peritoneal dialysis without complications

INTERVENTIONS

Equipment/Supplies

- Dialysate solution in 250 ml, 500 ml, or 1 L containers with prescribed dextrose and electrolyte composition/concentration
- Administration set with cap, spike cover, and clamp
- Drainage tubing and containers or bag
- Bag and belt for CAPD

- Sterile dressings, gloves, antiseptic swabs for site dressing
- Sterile articles for starting and discontinuing procedure
- Culture tube
- Disposable bag

Resident

- Explain the purpose of procedure and expected results
- Place in sitting or semi-Fowler's position and drape for privacy

✎ PROCEDURE

1. Perform handwashing.
2. Become familiar with dialysate concentration and amount, if IPD or CAPD administration, frequency of IPD, vital signs, I&O.
3. Prepare solution and supplies:
   a. Assemble the solution, set-up with tubing, clamp, cap, adapter, spike cover, empty bag and tubing, belt depending on type of dialysis.
   b. Warm the dialysate to body temperature (98.6°F) with a warm water bath or commercial warmer.
   c. Remove tubing and spike covers from the dialysate container(s) and connect the tubing, containers and the adapter to the tubing, hang the bags four feet above the site on a pole in close proximity to the resident and remove the air from the tubing.
   d. Maintain sterility of the line and the adapter that is to be connected to the peritoneal catheter.
4. Prepare and dress the peritoneal catheter site:
   a. Assemble sterile dressings, drape, antiseptic swabs on a sterile field.
   b. Put on gloves and remove dressings that cover the catheter and site, avoid touching catheter tip; discard the gloves and dressings.
   c. Note the dressing drainage and condition of the skin at the insertion site for redness, edema, crusting, pain.
   d. Put on sterile gloves and cleanse the catheter tip with antiseptic swabs and wrap the tip in a 4x4 with antiseptic.
   e. Cleanse catheter and site with a circular motion from the site outward and the catheter from the site to the tip with long strokes using a new antiseptic swab for each motion or stroke.
   f. Position the sterile fenestrated drape around the site with the catheter through the opening.
   g. Uncap the catheter and connect to the tubing from the dialysis set-up that contains the adapter, cover the connection with a dry dressing.
   h. Remove the drape, cleanse the site and apply dry dressings, coil the catheter under the dressing and tape in place.
   i. Proceed with the dialysis procedure.
5. Perform manual peritoneal dialysis:
   a. Place the empty drainage bags lower than the catheter site in close proximity to the resident.
   b. Following connection of the dialysate tubing to the catheter, begin the inflow phase allowing 10-20 minutes for completion, if pain is experienced, slow the inflow rate.
   c. Clamp and if another bag is to be infused, unclamp and allow another 10-20 minutes for inflow completion of the second bag.
   d. Clamp the tubing when the inflow phase has been completed and allow for dwell time of 30 minutes for IPD depending on orders and evaluation of the laboratory tests.
   e. If CAPD is being performed, connect an empty solution bag and wrap around the waist held in place by a belt; dwell time is usually 4-6 hours.
   f. Following inflow time, attach the catheter and tubing to the empty bags and allow for outflow phase to begin and complete in 20 minutes.
   g. If CAPD is being performed, unroll the bag at the waist, position below the catheter site and allow the outflow of the dialysate from the peritoneal cavity.
   h. Repeat the procedure at ordered frequency whether intermittent or continuous, connect new containers of dialysate and change tubing daily if the dialysis is continuous.
   i. If intermittent, redress the site at the completion of the dialysis as outlined in the site and catheter preparation in this procedure and cover with a transparent occlusive dressing.
   j. Note the characteristics of the outflow (color, cloudiness) or an outflow that is greater than the inflow.
   k. Pour the effluent obtained from the outflow down the drain.

6. Dispose of used articles and supplies from any of the procedures using Universal Precautions.

❧ PROBLEM-SOLVING ACTIONS

1. Use a mask and strict sterile technique when performing this procedure as the resident is at risk for infection.

2. Vital signs should be taken prior to and every 15 minutes during the procedure to evaluate for excessive fluid loss or retention.

3. Monitor laboratory tests such as creatinine, blood, urea nitrogen, glucose, proteins, and electrolytes to determine renal function and concentrations and components of the dialysate.

4. Perform other daily care during the outflow phase when abdominal distention is minimized.

5. Medications can be added to the dialysate to prevent infection (antibiotic), obstruction (heparin), electrolyte imbalance (potassium), pain (lidocaine).

❧ EVALUATION

Safe and correct intermittent or continuous peritoneal dialysis, absence of skin breakdown or infection at the site or complications associated with any phase of the dialysis procedure.

TOILETING, BEDPAN/URINAL

The bedpan and urinal are toileting devices used for urination and/or defecation by individuals who are confined to bed and not able or permitted to use bathroom facilities. The containers provide an accurate measurement of output and collection of a urine or feces specimen for testing and assessment of waste products. The focus of this procedure is to assist the male to use the urinal and bedpan and the female to use the bedpan in privacy and with comfort.

ASSESSMENT

Usual pattern (frequency and time) of voiding and defecation, history of presence of disorders causing urinary and bowel elimination abnormalities, signs and symptoms of urinary or bowel dysfunction, bowel sounds, bladder distention, ability to carry out self-care in toileting

NURSING DIAGNOSES

Impaired Physical Mobility; Self-Care Deficit, Toileting, Altered Urinary Elimination Patterns, Anxiety

GOAL

Bowel and urinary elimination provided with use of bedpan and urinal

INTERVENTIONS

Equipment/Supplies

- Individual bedpan, regular or fracture type
- Individual urinal
- Toilet tissue
- Wash cloth, towel, soap and warm water in a basin

- Protective pad
- Deodorizer
- Talcum powder
- Disposable gloves

Resident

- Place in semi-Fowler's position for female and male on a bedpan, high-Fowler's or standing position for male using urinal
- Explain purpose of procedure and expected results

- Pull curtain or close door for privacy, cover if needed

PROCEDURE

1. Perform handwashing.
2. Become familiar with ability for self-toileting and amount of assistance needed for bedpan or urinal use, need for I&O monitoring or specimen collection, pattern of urinary and bowel elimination (on arising and before sleep, before meals and treatments/procedures).
3. Maintain individual utensils and avoid sharing these with other residents.
4. Rinse metal utensils with warm water before using, lightly sprinkle talcum on bedpan edges to place and remove easier without friction on the skin.

5. Place the utensil within reach on the bed.
6. Provide a urinal for urinary elimination:
   a. Lift a portion of the covers and hand the urinal to the resident to position or place the urinal in between the legs with the bottom lower than the open top and lift the penis into the urinal.
   b. Allow time to void in privacy, gently shake the penis to remove urine after voiding and remove urinal from its position without spilling.
   c. Allow to stand at the side of the bed to void with support if difficult to void lying down, hold the urinal in place if necessary.
   d. Provide a damp cloth to wash hands.
   e. Take urinal to bathroom, empty it, rinse, replace in proper storage place.
7. Provide a bedpan for urinary/bowel elimination:
   a. Fold back the top linens on one side and request to flex knees and raise buttocks, assist with hand under the small of the back.
   b. Place the bedpan under the buttocks in proper position, replace covers, raise head of bed to a comfortable position for elimination, place toilet tissue within reach.
   c. If unable to raise hips or lift, position on the side and place the bedpan against the buttocks in the proper position and turn to position on the back while holding the bedpan in position, adjust for proper position, replace covers, raise head of bed to comfortable position for elimination, place toilet tissue within reach.
   d. Remove bedpan by lowering the bed, fold top linens back, request to lift hips or assist by placing hand under small of back and, with dominant hand, remove the bedpan and place on chair or bed.
   e. Turn on side and cleanse genitalia wiping from front to back and/or anus with toilet tissue and wash with soap and water and dry, depending on what is needed.
   f. Offer damp washcloth and small towel to clean hands.
   g. Remove bedpan to bathroom, empty and cleanse, store for future use.
8. Note characteristics of urine and feces, measure urine and record if I&O is being monitored, collect specimen if needed.
9. Use deodorant in the room if necessary or appropriate to control odors.

❧ PROBLEM-SOLVING ACTIONS

1. Use gloves to perform these procedures to prevent transmission of micro-organisms.
2. Allow as much independence in the use of a urinal or bedpan and cleansing following elimination as possible.
3. Apply a skin protector ointment to anus following defecation and cleansing if diarrhea or irritation is present.
4. Linens that become wet or soiled should be changed.
5. Raise the head of the bed to a height most conducive to elimination.

❧ EVALUATION

Daily elimination in urinal and/or bedpan with ease and comfort at time and frequency of usual pattern.

TOILETING, COMMODE/BATHROOM

T*he commode is a chair containing an opening similar to a toilet seat that allows for a pan or bucket to slide in under the opening to receive urine or feces. It is placed near the bed and used as an alternative to the bedpan and bathroom when it is possible for a resident to get out of bed but not able to be independent and mobile enough to go to the bathroom. Like the toilet in the bathroom, the commode allows the resident to assume the more normal sitting position for elimination by the female and defecation by the male. The bathroom is the facility used when the resident is capable of complete self-care in toileting.*

❧ ASSESSMENT

Usual pattern of elimination, ability to provide own toileting needs, difficulty in using a bedpan for elimination, urinary or bowel abnormalities

❧ NURSING DIAGNOSES

High Risk for Impaired Skin Integrity; Self-Care Deficit, Toileting; Altered Urinary Elimination Patterns; Diarrhea; High Risk for Trauma

❧ GOALS

Bowel and urinary elimination provided with use of bedside commode or toilet in the bathroom

❧ INTERVENTIONS

Equipment/Supplies

- Commode
- Toilet tissue
- Wash cloth, towel, soap and warm water
- Deodorizer
- Bath blanket
- Disposable gloves

Resident

- Explain purpose for procedure and expected results
- Pull curtain or close room or bathroom door if desired
- Place in sitting position on the commode or toilet
- Place bath blanket over legs for privacy and warmth

❧ PROCEDURE

1. Perform handwashing.
2. Become familiar with ability to perform toileting procedures independently or amount of assistance needed, type of toileting facility to be used, need for I&O monitoring or specimen collection, pattern of daily bowel and urinary elimination.
3. Maintain privacy and place toilet tissue within reach.
4. Provide for bathroom toileting:
   a. Assist with robe and slippers if needed.
   b. Assist to bathroom (walk or wheelchair), advise to use holding bars to walk, assume sitting position on toilet, and getting up from toilet.
   c. Assist with cleansing following elimination if needed and to use sink to wash hands.
   d. Assist to return to bed and remove robe and slippers if needed.

5. Provide a commode for toileting:
   a. Place commode parallel to the bed and lock wheels if present.
   b. Open cover over opening in seat of the commode.
   c. Assist to sit at the side of the bed and then stand, pivot to seat on the commode in a comfortable position, cover with the bath blanket if needed.
   d. Provide toilet tissue within reach or assist to cleanse including washing and drying the anal area following elimination.
   e. Offer damp wash cloth and towel to clean hands.
   f. Assist to stand and return to bed to a position of comfort.
   g. Close lid on commode, remove the pan or roll the commode to the bathroom and empty, rinse and cleanse the pan, return for future use.

6. Note characteristics of urine and feces before emptying the commode pan or flushing the toilet, measure urine and record if I&O is being monitored, collect specimen if needed.

7. Use deodorizer in room or bathroom if needed or appropriate to control odors.

✌ PROBLEM-SOLVING ACTIONS

1. Encourage to use holding bars in bathroom to prevent falls.

2. Gloves should be worn to cleanse perineal area.

3. A raised toilet seat can be helpful for those who have difficulty getting on or off the toilet.

4. Encourage self-care in toileting as this promotes comfort, self-esteem and privacy.

5. Disinfect commode or toilet seat if contaminated with feces.

✌ EVALUATION

Daily elimination in commode or toilet with or without assistance at time and frequency of usual pattern.

URINARY DIVERSION MANAGEMENT

Urinary diversions are surgically-created urostomies to provide a system of urine drainage via the abdominal surface (cutaneous ureterostomy) or into a loop of the ileus or colon portion of the bowel (ileal conduit, ileal bladder conduit, vesicostomy). The urine flows from the conduit or reservoir created by the surgery to a stoma situated on the abdominal wall and can be temporary or permanent depending on the reason for the diversion. A diversion is performed to accommodate urinary elimination in those with a neurogenic bladder, malignant tumor of the bladder, chronic urinary tract infections, or trauma to the urinary bladder. The management of urinary diversion includes the application, removal, emptying and cleansing of the drainage appliance, peristomal care, prevention of skin irritation, appliance leakage and odor, and provision of support and assistance in achieving independence in the care of the stoma. A vesicostomy does not require an appliance but is created to allow for periodic removal of urine from the bladder pouch created by surgery (see Catheterization, Intermittent Urethral/Suprapubic/Continent Vesicostomy). Clean technique is utilized in the performance of procedures associated with urinary diversion care.

ASSESSMENT

Type and reason for urinary diversion, stoma for color, edema, pain, peristomal skin for redness, excoriation, breaks, pouch for leakage or odor, urinary flow and characteristics, timing and frequency of emptying or changing of appliance

NURSING DIAGNOSES

High Risk for Impaired Skin Integrity; Ineffective Individual Coping; High Risk for Infection; Altered Urinary Elimination Patterns

GOALS

Continuous drainage of urine via urinary diversion with appropriate care of stoma and performance of urine collection procedures, peristomal skin intact and free of irritation

INTERVENTIONS

Equipment/Supplies

- Appliance, disposable or reusable
- Skin barrier, sealant, adhesive, paste
- Appliance belt
- Gauze dressings and tape
- Basin with warm water, soap, towel
- Disposable gloves
- Scissors, measuring device
- Disposable bag for used articles
- Calibrated measuring recepticle
- Protective pads
- Deodorizer

Resident

- Explain purpose for procedure and expected results
- Place in supine or other position of comfort, semi-Fowler's or sitting

❧ PROCEDURE

1. Perform handwashing.

2. Become familiar with specific procedures to be performed, type of diversion and ability for and extent of self-care, need for I&O monitoring, effect on body image and self-esteem.

3. Assemble supplies needed for procedures to be performed and provide privacy during care.

4. Place protective pads under the buttocks to protect bed linens.

5. Perform appliance emptying:
   a. Put on gloves.
   b. Empty pouch by opening the drain cap or valve and allow the urine to flow into a calibrated container, note amount and characteristics.
   c. Place deodorant in the pouch and replace the drain valve.
   d. Empty when the pouch is ⅔ full to prevent pulling on the appliance from the weight of the urine that can cause leakage around the appliance.

6. Perform removal of the appliance:
   a. Put on gloves.
   b. Empty the pouch (see above) and remove the belt if one is worn.
   c. Gently lift the faceplate or wafer part of the appliance while pushing skin down and away from the stoma, avoid peeling it from the skin.
   d. Cleanse the stoma with warm water and soft cloth and cover with a toilet tissue or tampon while cleansing the skin.
   e. Cleanse the peristomal skin with special cleansing preparation and warm water and pat dry.
   f. Apply the moisture skin barrier, ointment, cream or other preparation.
   g. Wash appliance, dry and store or discard according to universal precautions.

7. Perform application of appliance:
   a. Put on gloves, add deodorant to the pouch to be applied.
   b. Measure the stoma and cut the proper size hole in the disk or wafer, apply karaya powder or other treatment to the skin if it is irritated.
   c. Apply the disk or wafer around the stoma and press firmly around the edges.
   d. Use skin paste to fill any areas between the stoma and barrier.
   e. Remove the cover from the barrier and peel the paper backing from the adhesive ring on the pouch.
   f. Place the opening over the stoma and apply a firm pressure to the seal.
   g. If a barrier is not used, place the opening of the pouch on the skin sealant and allow to set.
   h. Attach belt and connect the tubing to a closed drainage system or leg bag if desired.

8. Store cleansed, reusable appliances in clean plastic bags for future use.

❧ PROBLEM-SOLVING ACTIONS

1. Skin assessment and care at the device site should be performed with each appliance removal.

2. Maintain drainage tube patency when attached to a drainage system.

3. A drainage system to a large collection bag can be used at night to avoid the need to disturb the resident's sleep by emptying the pouch.

4. Appliance can vary from temporary or permanent and procedures for removal and application will vary with type used, information inserts that accompany the appliance should be followed.

5. All urine emptied from the pouches or drainage systems should be measured if I&O is being monitored.

❧ EVALUATION

Daily correct and effective management of all aspects of urinary diversion care, peristomal skin intact and free from irritation.

URINARY INCONTINENCE MANAGEMENT

Urinary incontinence is the inability to control the passage of urine. Incontinence may be a total involuntary or partial emptying of the bladder. It is the result of an interference with the sphincter muscle control that is caused by a neuromuscular condition, weak musculature, medication regimen that affects the consciousness of the urge to void, and renal/urologic disorders such as tumors and infection. Incontinence management includes procedures such as bladder retraining, the application of external devices or incontinence collectors (both male and female) maintenance of skin integrity, and preservation of self-esteem by preventing the embarrassment and dependence caused by the loss of control. Urinary incontinence in the elderly can often be the result of the inability to reach the bathroom in time or the lack of attention and assistance from the staff.

⊱ ASSESSMENT

Age, general health status and medical conditions contributing to incontinence, medications that affect awareness or orientation, ability to use the bedpan, urinal, commode or bathroom, usual elimination pattern, skin condition for irritation or breaks

⊱ NURSING DIAGNOSES

Incontinence, Functional, Reflex, or Total; High Risk for Impaired Skin Integrity; Self-Care Deficit, Toileting; Altered Pattern of Urinary Elimination

⊱ GOALS

State of maximum urinary continence achieved with avoidance of complications

⊱ INTERVENTIONS

Equipment/Supplies

- External female urinary collection device
- External male urinary catheter (sheath or condom)
- Adhesive or other fastening material

- Incontinence pants, pads
- Protective pads for bed

- Bedpan, urinal, commode, toilet tissue

- Damp washcloth, warm water, towel
- Clean linen as needed

- Protective skin ointment, spray, wipes

- Deodorizer
- Disposable gloves

Resident

- Explain purpose for procedure and expected results

- Place in supine or sidelying position for urinary device application

⊱ PROCEDURE

1. Perform handwashing.

2. Become familiar with urinary continence status, cause of incontinence, pattern of elimination, retraining potential, use of devices.

3. Provide urinary incontinence care:
   a. Assemble cleansing articles, protective pads and briefs, gloves, clean linens.
   b. Remove top linens and cover with a bath blanket.
   c. If briefs in place, untape and lower between legs.
   d. Place in sidelying position, roll bottom soiled linen against back and place towel over the rolled linens.
   e. Wash the area with mild soap and warm water, rinse, pat dry.
   f. Apply skin protector, ointment or other prescribed treatment.
   g. Place the clean briefs in position on the back, turn to a supine position, bring the front of the briefs up to the waist and attach in place, and move to the side of the bed.
   h. Remove the soiled linen and bring the clean bottom linen from under the resident and tuck in both sides.
   i. Use siderails to protect from falls on opposite side of giving care.
   j. Remove bath blanket and replace top linens, place in position of comfort.

4. Provide urinary incontinence management:
   a. Assemble bedpan, urinal, commode to use, other supplies needed for procedure.
   b. Remind to void or provide an opportunity to void every 2 hours whether need is felt or not, adjust time schedule to fluid intake and usual pattern of urination.
   c. Provide privacy during urination, do not rush resident to perform.
   d. Apply a gentle pressure over the bladder area or use other methods to stimulate voiding, such as running water, placing hands in water.
   e. Offer fluids to total 2L/24 hours with a glass of fluid 30 minutes prior to the voiding attempt, avoid fluids before bedtime.
   f. Allow to wear incontinence pads between voidings.
   g. Increase interval between voiding as training improves, adjust schedule to meet changes in pattern.
   h. Maintain the schedule or modify until continence is established or utilize other methods of incontinence management if unsuccessful.

5. Apply external devices to female for urinary incontinence:
   a. Place in lithotomy position and drape for privacy.
   b. Cleanse and dry the perineal area to prepare for application of the device.
   c. Cut the faceplate to fit the area, remove the cover on the adhesive and place firmly around the genitalia, press the edges to the skin.
   d. Close the cap on the bag and open only to empty the pouch when needed or attach the tubing from a drainage device to the pouch opening (this will depend on the type of device used).
   e. Attach a urinary drainage system bag with straps or adhesive to a position of comfort on the thigh.
   f. When removing the device, gently peel off while holding the skin and replace if needed.
   g. Device can be washed, dried and reused, deodorant can be used in the collection system.

6. Apply external urinary devices to male for urinary incontinence:
   a. Place in a supine or sitting position and drape for privacy.
   b. Wash, rinse, and dry the penis to prepare for application of condom or sheath catheter.
   c. For a device that has an adhesive anchoring on the inside, remove the paper from the flexible adhesive strip and wrap around the penis in spiral fashion without overlapping ends.
   d. Roll the device outward and onto the penis and leave at least 2 inches between the tip of the penis and end of the device, press the device against the penis and adhesive strip and hold for 1 minute.
   e. Anchor the outside of the device with application of an adhesive strip in a spiral fashion described above.
   f. Attach the end of the device to a tubing and drainage bag that can hang on the bed or be strapped to the thigh.
   g. Remove the device and wash the penis daily and expose to air.
   h. Empty drainage bag as needed, cleanse and disinfect daily, use deodorizer in the bag when needed.

PROBLEM-SOLVING ACTIONS

1. Assessment of the skin under the device should be performed with each removal or change.

2. Skin protection can be applied during device changes.

3. Apply the external device snugly but without constriction to the circulation.

4. Maintain drainage tube patency to prevent urine accumulation in the device and possible displacement and leakage.

5. Shave hair if needed to accommodate secure application of the device.

6. An improvised device can be constructed using a regular condom that has a hole punctured at the end of it and placed in a piece of tubing, held in place with a rubber band and positioned on the penis.

EVALUATION

Daily progress in continence retraining with an increased sense of control of urinary pattern, correct and effective use of external urinary collection devices.

UNIT XI

GASTROINTESTINAL PROCEDURES

- Bowel Diversion Management
- Bowel Incontinence Management
- Enemas
- Fecal Impaction Removal
- Feeding, Assistive/Complete
- Gastrostomy Tube Management
- Nasogastric Tube Management
- Total Parenteral Nutrition

BOWEL DIVERSION MANAGEMENT

Bowel diversions are surgically-created ostomies from the small or large intestinal tract (ileostomy or colostomy) to provide a system of drainage or for the removal of feces. The artificial opening or stoma on the abdominal surface is created to treat cancer, bowel obstruction, bowel inflammatory disease, and diverticulitis. It may be temporary or permanent. Its location depends on the disease or abnormality treated, and the drainage can be liquid, semisolid, or solid, depending on the site of the stoma. The most liquid comes from the ileum, the semisolid from the ascending and transverse colon, and the most solid from the descending colon. The management of bowel diversion includes the application, removal, emptying and cleansing of the drainage appliance, peristomal care, prevention of skin irritation, appliance leakage and odor, irrigation of a colostomy, and provision of support and assistance in achieving independence in the care of the stoma. A continent ileostomy or ileal reservoir is a pouch created from part of the ileum with a stoma at the abdominal surface and does not require an appliance. It is created to allow for periodic removal of drainage from the ileum pouch by intermittent catheterization. Clean technique is utilized in the performance of procedures associated with bowel diversion care.

❧ ASSESSMENT

Type and reason for bowel diversion, stoma for color, edema, pain, peristomal skin for redness, excoriation, breaks, pouch from appliance for leakage and characteristics of drainage or feces, timing and frequency of irrigation, emptying or changing of appliance

❧ NURSING DIAGNOSES

High Risk for Impaired Skin Integrity; Ineffective Individual Coping; Body Image Disturbance; Diarrhea; Constipation; Self-Care Deficit, Toileting

❧ GOALS

Continuous or intermittent drainage via bowel diversion without complications, correct and proper care of stoma, skin, and collection procedures

❧ INTERVENTIONS

Equipment/Supplies

- Appliance, disposable or reusable with all necessary parts, belt (temporary or permanent), stoma measuring device
- Disposable or reusable irrigation set with bag, tubing, clamp, cone tip, or catheter with guard, irrigating sheath, ostomy bag, and lubricant
- Irrigation fluid
- Disposable gloves
- Bedpan for irrigation
- Deodorant for appliance, room

- Skin barrier (disc or wafer), skin sealant (spray or wipe), skin adhesive (cement), skin paste, skin cream or gel
- Dressings and tape

- Catheter sets to drain ileal pouch with lubricant, receptacle, dressings, tape
- Basin of warm water, washcloth, towel
- Protective pads

<u>Resident</u>

- Explain purpose of procedure and expected results

- Place in supine or position for comfort, can be semi Fowler or sitting position depending upon the procedure

- Drape for privacy

❧ PROCEDURE

1. Perform handwashing.

2. Become familiar with specific procedures to be performed, type and location of diversion, ability to care for and extent of self-care, effect on body image and self esteem, adjustment to the bowel and stoma

3. Assemble the supplies needed for the procedures to be performed and set up within reach.

4. Place protective pads on bed where appropriate to protect linens.

5. Perform appliance removal or emptying:
   a. Put on disposable gloves.
   b. Empty ileostomy pouch of liquid drainage by opening the drain cap or unclamping the bottom and allowing the fluid to drain into a calibrated container, note amount and characteristics.
   c. Flush the pouch from the bottom opening with a squirt bottle of water, clamp or close the drain cap.
   d. Empty the pouch 4 to 5 times/day or when it is ⅔ full to prevent pulling on the appliance from the weight of the drainage as this can cause leakage around the application site.
   e. Discard the pouch if disposable or wash, dry, and store if a reusable pouch.
   f. If the appliance is to be changed, remove the belt if one is worn.
   g. Gently lift the faceplate or wafer part of the appliance while pushing down and away from the stoma.
   h. Cleanse the stoma with warm water and a soft cloth.
   i. Cleanse the peristomal skin with special cleansing preparation and warm water, pat dry.
   j. Apply a skin barrier, ointment, gel, cream, or other preparation to the peristomal area.
   k. Dispose of supplies using Universal Precautions; cleanse, disinfect, and store reusable supplies.

6. Perform appliance application:
   a. Put on gloves, add deodorant to pouch if needed and place pin hole in the top of the bag to allow gas to escape.
   b. Measure the stoma and cut the proper size hole in the wafer or disk.
   c. Apply a skin sealant if skin is intact and not using an appliance with a sealant ring.
   d. Place the wafer or disk around the stoma and gently press it firmly to the skin.
   e. Use skin paste to fill in areas between stoma and the barrier.
   f. If skin is irritated, apply karaya powder or paste to absorb moisture and protect the skin from further damage.
   g. If a one piece system is used, remove paper backing from the adhesive on the pouch and covering from the barrier and attach the opening over the stoma; if a barrier is not used, apply directly on a skin sealant.
   h. Attach a belt if used.
   i. Cleanse, disinfect, store reusable appliance in a clean plastic bag.

7. Perform colostomy irrigation:
   a. Put on gloves.
   b. Prepare solution, usually about 1000 ml of tap water at 105° F, in the container and hang 12-18 inches above the level of the stoma.
   c. Connect the catheter in a cone tip to the tubing and expel the air; clamp the tubing.
   d. Seat on the toilet, commode, or at the side of the bed with a bedpan on a chair below the stoma level and drape the legs.
   e. Remove the pouch appliance and discard or save for later cleansing and reuse.
   f. Cleanse the stoma and peristomal skin with a special cleansing agent and allow to air dry.
   g. Peel the paper backing off the adhesive on the sleeve and apply the opening over the stoma, support with a belt if needed.
   h. Place the open end of the sleeve into the bedpan or toilet.
   i. Carefully insert the lubricated catheter 2-4 inches into the stoma, avoid using any force.

    j.   Hold the catheter and cone in place and pull the top of the sleeve around the tube to prevent splashing of fluid.

    k.   Unclamp the tubing and allow the water to flow at a rate that would take 15 minutes to instill all but 500 ml of water, stop if cramping occurs and start again.

    l.   After fluid has been instilled, clamp tubing and remove cone tip or catheter.

    m. Allow 15 minutes for the fluid to return into the toilet or bedpan, run the remaining 500 ml of water through the top of the sleeve to clear it of feces.

    n.   Remove the lower open part from the bedpan or toilet, clamp it and fold up and attach to the top of the sleeve; leave for 30 minutes to collect any additional amounts of return.

    o.   Detach the sleeve, rinse with water from a container poured through the top of the sleeve until clear of all feces.

    p.   Clamp tubing, gently remove the tip, sleeve and belt.

    q.   Wash, rinse, and dry peristomal area and reapply a change of appliance if needed or a change of appliance pouch.

    r.   Wash, disinfect, rinse, and store reusable irrigation supplies in a clean plastic bag for future use; use room deodorant as needed.

8. Return to a position of comfort following the procedure and note any adverse responses.

9. Perform continent ileostomy catheterization/care:

    a.   Put on gloves.

    b.   Position on the toilet or at the side of the bed.

    c.   Remove any dressings/tape and discard, note condition of stoma, gently wash with saline and a sponge.

    d.   Lubricate the catheter tip with water or water soluble lubricant and gently insert it 2 inches into the stoma or until resistance is met.

    e.   Allow to drain in the bedpan/toilet, usually 10 minutes depending upon the consistency of the drainage.

    f.   If drainage clogs the catheter, irrigate with a catheter tipped 50 ml syringe containing 30 ml of water; remove the catheter and reinsert another if the irrigation does not clear it.

    g.   Remove the catheter, cleanse the stoma and peristomal area, apply skin protector cream, gel, or other barrier ointment.

    h.   Wash, disinfect, rinse the catheters and allow to dry, store for future use, discard other used articles according to Universal Precautions.

❧ PROBLEM-SOLVING ACTIONS

1. Skin assessment and care at the diversion site should be performed with each appliance removal.

2. Appliances vary in styles from one-piece to two-piece for temporary use to a permanent faceplate to hold the appliance in place.

3. Ileostomy pouches can be worn for up to 7 days without changing but with regular emptying; the best times are before meals and bedtime.

4. Allow and encourage as much independence in performing the procedures as possible while still supporting and assisting when needed.

5. Complaints of itching or burning under the appliance should result in removal for skin assessment immediately.

6. Pouches are usually odor proof, but can also have a deodorant added.

7. Persistent leakage or poorly fitted appliances can cause injury to the stoma and skin breakdown, a stoma can change in size and shape, measurements and appliance application should reflect this.

8. Assist to make dietary selections that do not cause diarrhea, constipation or those that are gas forming.

9. Information and directions for use of ostomy products are provided by the manufacturer and should always be consulted before using.

❧ EVALUATION

Effective drainage of feces removal via bowel diversion at appropriate times and utilizing proper technique, peristomal skin intact and free from irritation

BOWEL INCONTINENCE MANAGEMENT

Bowel incontinence is the inability to control the passage of feces and occurs with an absence of voluntary control of the sphincters of the rectum that results in spontaneous elimination or fecal loss. It can be caused by any condition that affects anal sphincter function such as neurological disorder, fistula, infection, fissure, diarrhea, or medication regimens that affect the urge to defecate. Bowel incontinence management includes rehabilitation with rectal retraining, the application of external devices or collectors, maintenance of skin integrity, and preservation of self esteem by preventing embarrassment and dependence.

ASSESSMENT

General health status and medical conditions contributing to fecal incontinence, medication regimen, skin condition for irritation or breaks, awareness of urge to defecate

NURSING DIAGNOSES

Bowel Incontinence; High Risk for Impaired Skin Integrity, Self-Care Deficit, Toileting

GOAL

State of maximum bowel continence achieved with avoidance of complications

INTERVENTIONS

Equipment/Supplies

- Fecal incontinence collector
- Incontinence pants or pads
- Protective pads for bed
- Bedpan, commode, toilet tissue
- Soap, warm water, towel, washcloth
- Clean linen as needed
- Protective skin ointment, spray, wipes
- Deodorizer
- Disposable gloves

Resident

- Explain purpose for procedure and expected results
- Place in supine or sidelying position for fecal device application

PROCEDURE

1. Perform handwashing.
2. Become familiar with fecal continence status, cause of incontinence, pattern of defecation, retraining potential, use of collection device.
3. Provide fecal incontinence care:
   a. Assemble cleansing articles, protective pads and briefs, gloves, clean linens.
   b. Remove top linens and cover with a bath blanket.
   c. If briefs are in place, untape and lower between the legs.
   d. Place in sidelying position, cleanse feces with tissue.
   e. Roll bottom soiled linens against the back and place a towel under the back.
   f. Wash the area with mild soap and warm water, rinse, pat dry.
   g. Apply skin protector, ointment or other prescribed treatment for skin care.

    h. Place the clean briefs in position at the back of the resident, turn to a supine position, bring the front of the briefs up to the waist, move the resident to the side of the bed.

    i. Remove the soiled bottom linen and bring the clean linen from under the resident, tuck in on both sides.

    j. Use side rails on the opposite side of giving care to protect from falls.

    k. Remove bath blanket and replace top linens, place in position of comfort.

    l. Dispose of soiled briefs using Universal Precautions.

4. Provide bowel management:

    a. Assemble bedpan, commode, and other supplies needed for the procedure.

    b. Select time of day, preferably after breakfast if possible, and provide a warm beverage prior to defecation time.

    c. Administer a suppository 30 minutes prior to the selected time.

    d. Apply digital stimulation to the anus or administer a small volume enema prior to defecation.

    e. Assist to use bedpan, commode or the bathroom and suggest to lean forward and bear down without straining to initiate defecation.

    f. Allow privacy and time for elimination, provide tissues for cleansing or assist in cleansing if defecation successful, assist to wash hands.

    g. Repeat the procedure for at least 3 days and modify to suit resident if needed, offer praise for attempts as well as successes.

5. Apply external devices to female or male for bowel incontinence:

    a. Place in sidelying position and drape for privacy.

    b. Cleanse and dry the perianal area to prepare for application of the device.

    c. Cut the faceplate to fit the area, remove the cover on the adhesive, and firmly place around the anal area, press the edges against skin to secure.

    d. Check to be sure that there are no openings in the pouch if a one-time disposable pouch or that the opening is clamped closed if a reusable pouch, place a deodorant in the pouch.

    e. When removing the device, gently peel off while holding the skin and replace when needed.

    f. Wash device, dry, and store, for reuse depending on type.

PROBLEM-SOLVING ACTIONS

1. Assessment of the skin under the device should be performed with each removal or change.

2. Shave hair if needed to accommodate secure application of the device.

EVALUATION

Daily progress in fecal continence management with an increased sense of control of bowel elimination pattern, correct and effective use of external fecal collection devices

ENEMAS

*E*nemas introduce fluid into the rectum and colon via the anus. They are administered to cleanse the lower bowel to relieve constipation and flatulence, prepare the bowel for diagnostic procedures, administer medications, and to assist in bowel retraining to correct fecal incontinence. In one type of enema, a large volume of solution is instilled with a flexible tube and container of tap water, soapy water or saline solution for cleansing purposes. Another type of enema is administered by the instillation of small volumes of solution with a short, firm plastic tip attached to a commercially-prepared phosphate solution (Fleet) for cleansing, or oil retention to soften the feces prior to elimination. Clean technique is utilized for the performance of these procedures.

✇ ASSESSMENT

Reason for enema (constipation, incontinence and retraining, fecal impaction, flatulence), type of enema, usual bowel elimination pattern, use of laxatives, feces characteristics

✇ NURSING DIAGNOSES

Bowel Incontinence; Constipation; Self-Care Deficit, Toileting

✇ GOAL

Maintenance of optimal bowel elimination pattern with or without the administration of enemas

✇ INTERVENTIONS

Equipment/Supplies

- Enema container or bag with tubing and rectal tube, pole to hang it
- Toilet tissue, bedpan, commode
- Solution for large volume enema
- Protector pad
- Commercial phosphate or oil retention enema
- Disposable gloves
- Water soluble lubricant

Resident

- Explain the purpose of procedure and expected results
- Place in left sidelying position and drape for privacy

✇ PROCEDURE

1. Perform handwashing.
2. Become familiar with the type of enema and supplies needed.
3. Place protector pad under the buttocks; if bedpan is to be used, place on the bed within reach.
4. Administer large volume enema:
   a. Assemble the correct amount of solution (500-1000ml) in the container and check the temperature for 105° F; hang on a pole 12-18 inches above the buttocks and clear the tubing of air and clamp.
   b. Put on gloves.
   c. Lubricate the end of the tubing, separate the buttocks with the nondominant hand and observe the anus

for hemorrhoids or other conditions.

d. Hold the tube in the dominant hand and touch the tip to the anus to allow the anus to relax, request to breathe through the mouth.

e. Insert the tube 2-3 inches into the rectum in the direction of the umbilicus and past the internal sphincter muscle.

f. Release buttocks while holding the tube in the rectum, unclamp the tubing and allow the solution to flow by gravity (75-100 ml/minute is an ideal rate).

g. Allow at least 10 minutes for the solution to flow, slow rate or stop intermittently if resident is cramping or unable to retain the fluid.

h. Clamp and remove the tube when a small amount of solution remains or the resident cannot tolerate additional solution, hold the buttocks together if fluid cannot be retained.

i. Ask the resident to retain the solution for 5 minutes, or as long as possible, assist to the bathroom, commode, or on the bedpan with a supply of toilet tissue nearby.

j. Remove the enema supplies, cleanse and store for future use or discard according to Universal Precautions.

5. Administer small volume enema:

a. Assemble the commercially prepared enema or small volume of solution to be administered.

b. Put on gloves.

c. If a non-commercial small volume enema is given, introduce the catheter into the rectum and proceed as for large volume enema except reduce the rate of flow.

d. If a commercial Fleet type enema is given, remove from the box, remove the cover from the lubricated tip, add lubrication if needed.

e. Insert the tip into the rectum in the direction of the umbilicus.

f. Crush the container with slow, constant pressure until all possible solution is administered, remove and discard in the box container.

g. Request to retain the solution until cramping is felt if a cleansing type enema is given, longer or until fecal impaction is removed if a retention type enema is given.

h. Assist to the bathroom, commode, or on the bedpan and place toilet tissue within reach.

i. Discard used supplies using Universal Precautions.

6. Assist to wash hands and to comfortable position following defecation.

7. Use a room deodorant at the conclusion of the procedure.

❧ PROBLEM-SOLVING ACTIONS

1. If possible, administer an enema before mealtime.

2. Apply a rectal tube guard if sphincter control is not strong enough to retain fluid.

3. Inform of activity, fluid and food inclusions that can assist in defecation.

4. If pain or obstruction of tube insertion is experienced, withdraw the tube and notify the physician.

5. Provide assistance for those who are not functionally independent.

6. Offer as much privacy and support as possible because the procedure causes anxiety and embarrassment to many residents.

7. Failure to expel the solution requires removal by siphoning depending on agency policy.

8. If on enteric precautions, double bag and label all discarded supplies.

❧ EVALUATION

Relief of bowel elimination problems following enema administration

FECAL IMPACTION REMOVAL

*F*ecal impaction is the accumulation and retention of a mass of hardened stool in the rectum
that prevents normal bowel elimination. It is the result of constipation or drugs that cause
constipation, a failure to defecate over a period of time, or inadequate fluid intake or physical
activity. Impaction removal becomes necessary when other methods such as laxatives and
enemas fail to induce defecation. It is performed by breaking up the mass with digital
manipulation and manual removal of a small amount of the feces at a time.

ASSESSMENT

Bowel elimination pattern and last bowel movement, presence of hard feces determined by digital
examination, feeling of abdominal or rectal fullness, pain, anorexia, laxative or enema administration,
hemorrhoids or rectal abnormalities, loose or diarrheal feces

NURSING DIAGNOSES

High Risk for Impaired Tissue Integrity; Pain; Self-Care Deficit, Toileting; Constipation

GOALS

Safe, effective removal of fecal impaction and return to baseline bowel elimination pattern

INTERVENTIONS

Equipment/Supplies

- Bedpan
- Disposable gloves
- Water soluble lubricant
- Toilet tissue, cleansing wipes
- Protector pad

Resident

- Explain the purpose of procedure and expected results
- Place in sidelying position and drape for privacy

PROCEDURE

1. Perform handwashing.
2. Place the bedpan on the bed in close proximity.
3. Put glove on dominant hand and lubricate forefinger.
4. Insert the gloved finger into the rectum upward in the direction of the umbilicus.
5. Gently work the finger into the mass and break it into small pieces.
6. Remove each piece and place into the bedpan.
7. Continue until the impaction has been completely removed.
8. Remove glove and discard according to Universal Precautions.
9. Cleanse the anal area with tissue, soothing wipes, or warm water and washcloth, pat dry.
10. Remove bed protector and bedpan, dispose of feces according to Universal Precautions, cleanse and store the bedpan for future use.
11. Place in a comfortable position.

❧ PROBLEM-SOLVING ACTIONS

1. Request to take deep breaths when inserting finger into the anus and removing the feces to relax the sphincter.

2. Administer oil retention enema to soften feces prior to removal.

3. Stop the procedure if the resident is too fatigued or experiencing extreme pain and allow to rest before continuing.

4. Assess for changes in pulse, skin color, dizziness, faintness, diaphoresis and stop the procedure, observe for a reduction in the symptoms.

5. Administer cleansing enema following impaction removal if needed.

❧ EVALUATION

Fecal impaction removed without rectal or anal injury

FEEDING, ASSISTIVE/COMPLETE

*A*ssistive or complete feeding of meals is provided to residents who have decreased appetites or are unable to eat independently because of disabilities, confusion, weakness, or neuromuscular disorders. The process of eating fulfills the basic nutritional need and is a major factor in preventing illness and promoting wellness. Dietary requirements and feeding needs should be incorporated into resident preferences, cultural factors, illness, appetite, and functional abilities. Modifications in consistency and texture, often necessary for the elderly with chewing or swallowing problems, are also considered in dietary planning. The amount of assistance needed can vary or be temporary, as for an individual with a casted arm. The need can also be permanent as for those with paralysis or those who are sightless. It is important to allow and encourage as much independence in self-feeding as possible to enhance self-worth and provide optimal control of daily living activities. This can be accomplished for the permanently disabled by the use of assistive devices and techniques that stimulate chewing, sucking, and swallowing.

ASSESSMENT

Nutritional status including excesses and deficits, medications that affect appetite or nutritional intake, illness or condition that requires dietary restrictions or modifications, food allergies, weight gains or losses, need for rehabilitation, pain, anorexia, fatigue, nausea, problem with chewing/swallowing

NURSING DIAGNOSES

High Risk for Aspiration; Fatigue; Pain; Altered Nutrition: Less Than Body Requirements; Powerlessness; Self-Care Deficit, Feeding; Sensory/Perceptual Alterations, Gustatory, Olfactory; Impaired Swallowing

GOALS

Maximal participation in daily self-feeding, optimal nutritional intake with partial or complete assistance

INTERVENTIONS

Equipment/Supplies

- Tray containing diet (food and fluids)
- Napkin or hand towel
- Assistive devices
- Straws for fluids

Resident

- Position of comfort, usually high Fowler's in bed or sitting in a chair at a table

PROCEDURE

1. Perform handwashing.
2. Become familiar with diet and any special modifications, amount of assistance needed, interest in self feeding, nutritional assessment for history, pattern and other characteristics of food and fluid intake.
3. Provide a pleasant environment, remove odors and used equipment and supplies.

4. Provide oral care and an opportunity to wash hands with a damp cloth prior to eating; check if dentures are in place and fit properly.

5. Clear and wash the overbed or other table and position the correct tray in front of the resident.

6. Remove the covers on the hot food and allow to view the food.

7. Assist with feeding as needed:
    a. Place the napkin or small towel over the chest or tuck under the chin.
    b. Arrange the dishes and articles on the tray for convenience and easy access, remove and discard the wrappings.
    c. Spread the dishes on the tray to avoid spilling.
    d. Cut meat, place straw in glass, open and pour fluids from a container into a glass or cup, open salt, sugar, or pepper and use on food or in fluids as desired or requested.
    e. Supply assistive devices such as swivel spoons, built up or long handled utensils, plate guards, non-slip guard on glass, large handled mugs, suction cups on the dishes.
    f. Allow to place the food into the mouth with fingers or after placed on the utensil, hold the containers of fluid and allow to hold straw if able; check to be sure food is not too hot.
    g. If fatigued, provide more assistance in feeding; have the resident take a bite independently and then feed him or her a bite using another utensil.
    h. Always allow plenty of time for chewing and swallowing, avoid rushing as this can cause fatigue, refusal to continue eating, and choking.
    i. At the conclusion of the meal, allow to wash the hands and face and provide oral care.
    j. Remove the tray and note the amount of food and fluid ingested.

8. Perform complete feeding:
    a. Prepare the resident as for assistive feeding.
    b. Place a chair near the tray and sit facing the resident.
    c. Prepare the tray as for assistive feeding; check to be sure food is not too hot.
    d. Start with small amounts of food and wait before offering the next bite.
    e. Start with pureed foods and progress to soft and then solid foods as swallowing is established.
    f. Bring the food to the mouth at the chin level rather than the eye level.
    g. Assist with sucking by holding lips around the straw, with swallowing by holding the lips between the thumb and forefinger.
    h. Offer fluids during the feeding to lubricate the oral cavity and assist in swallowing efforts.
    i. Perform techniques to enhance chewing by tapping or stretching the masseter muscle, swallowing by stroking the sides of the larynx with the fingertips, sucking by tapping, stretching, or applying pressure to the muscles around the mouth, opening the mouth by touching the lips with the utensil, closing the mouth by applying pressure above or below the lips in an upward or downward direction.
    j. Conclude the meal as for assistive feeding.

9. Follow any feeding techniques developed by the therapist and maintain consistency in feeding. procedure.

❧ PROBLEM-SOLVING ACTIONS

1. Adjust the consistency of the food to fit the position when eating to prevent aspiration or choking.

2. Provide smaller, more frequent meals if intake is poor or appetite is reduced.

3. For a sightless resident, arrange the food in a familiar pattern and describe the foods and their placement, use the clock hours to identify the location of the foods such as meat at 3 o'clock, potato at 12 o'clock.

4. Lemon ice, sweet fluids can stimulate salivation, milk products can thicken secretions.

5. Avoid offering foods that are too hot or cold as this can affect the sense of taste.

❧ EVALUATION

Daily optimal fluid and food intake with as much independence or assistance necessary

GASTROSTOMY TUBE MANAGEMENT

A gastrostomy is a surgically-created abdominal opening into the stomach for the purpose of administering feedings. A stoma is created to allow for long-term feedings and can contain a button with a mushroom-type dome to secure the device under the skin and a plug that can be opened or closed at the surface of the skin. It can also contain an inflatable tube inserted into the stomach and skin disk to secure the position of the tube for the purpose of feedings. Another alternative is the intermittent insertion and removal of a tube into the stoma for intermittent feedings. The gastrostomy is performed and used for long term, intermittent and continuous liquid feedings to avoid the problems encountered in long term nasogastric tube feedings. Included in the management of a gastrostomy is the care of the stoma site, insertion and removal of the tube or button, and preparation and administration of the formula feedings via the gastrostomy. The gastrostomy button implantation is especially useful because it is easy to maintain, decreases site irritation, and is less likely to become displaced or develop leakage of the gastric contents as it contains an antireflux valve. For those who are able and willing, intermittent feedings via gastrostomy can be performed by the resident with or without assistance. Medications are also administered via the gastrostomy (see Medication, Nasogastric/Gastrostomy Tube). The clean technique is utilized in the feeding procedure with a combination of clean and sterile techniques in the care of the insertion site.

ASSESSMENT

Nutritional status, type of gastrostomy feeding device, amount, type, and frequency of liquid formula, insertion site for redness, edema, pain, drainage, breakdown, ability to perform the procedure and care for the gastrostomy

NURSING DIAGNOSES

High Risk for Impaired Skin Integrity; Self-Care Deficit, Feeding; High Risk for Infection; Ineffective Individual Coping; Altered Nutrition: Less Than Body Requirements

GOALS

Maintenance of nutritional status via gastrostomy feedings

INTERVENTIONS

Equipment/Supplies

- Feeding formula in a container or bag with tubing and connector
- Funnel or syringe barrel, water to clear tube
- Sterile dressings, antiseptic swabs, tape, ointment or skin protector
- Clean feeding tubes wrapped in a clean towel
- Disposable gloves

Resident

- Explain the purpose of procedure and expected results
- Place in semi-Fowler's position and drape for privacy

❧ PROCEDURE

1. Perform handwashing.

2. Become familiar with type of device, and feedings needed, amount of assistance needed.

3. Assemble the supplies needed for the procedures to be performed on a clean surface nearby.

4. Prepare the formula to be administered:
   a. Cleanse top of the can or bottle of formula, open and pour the correct amount into a measured feeding container; if refrigerated, allow to warm to room temperature before pouring into the container.
   b. Cover the container and place on the tray with the set-up or syringe for the administration of the formula by gravity.
   c. Label the remaining formula with the date and time and refrigerate to avoid using formula that has been opened and stored longer than 24 hours.
   d. If powdered formula is used, add contents to a liquid and mix well in a blender; if solid foods are to be given, blenderize into a liquid and add fluids to thin as needed.

5. Perform insertion and feeding via gastrostomy button:
   a. Put on gloves.
   b. Measure the stoma to determine the size of the button to insert.
   c. Place the lubricated obturator in the button and check the antireflux valve for patency.
   d. Lubricate the stoma and mushroom and gently insert into the stomach through the stoma.
   e. Carefully rotate and remove the obturator after the valve closes, check to be sure that the valve is closed and, if it sticks, reinsert the obturator until the valve closes.
   f. Close the flexible plug at the skin surface and allow to remain in place until feeding time.
   g. When administering a feeding, place the formula in a container with a tubing attached and clamp the tubing.
   h. Open the flexible plug and connect the tubing end to the adaptor on the button, allow the formula to flow into the stomach by gravity.
   i. Before the container empties, add 30-60 ml of water to clear tubing and ensure that all of the feeding enters the stomach.
   j. Disconnect the tubing from the adaptor and close the flexible plug.
   k. Remove the articles used, wash, dry and store for next feeding.

6. Perform insertion and feeding via a feeding tube:
   a. Put on gloves.
   b. Remove the dressing on the stoma and cleanse the area.
   c. To insert a balloon-type permanent gastrostomy tube, place a skin disk at the appropriate position on the abdomen, insert the tube into the opening up to the disk, inject distilled water in the appropriate amount to inflate the balloon, gently tug on the tube to ensure proper anchoring.
   d. Attach the syringe or tubing from a container of formula to the tube and allow to flow in by gravity
   e. Add 30 ml of water before the container is emptied to clear the tubing.
   f. Remove the syringe or container; cleanse, dry and store for next feeding, cap the tube and redress as needed.

7. Perform site or stoma care:
   a. Put on gloves and remove and discard the existing dressing and tape.
   b. Cleanse the skin area around the catheter or stoma with antiseptic swabs in a circular motion from the center outward using a new swab for each circle, follow with cleansing using saline sponges.
   c. Use a swab with normal saline to cleanse the stoma.
   d. Place a sterile gauze dressing on the stoma and tape.
   e. Place a sterile gauze dressing around the gastrostomy tube, position on another gauze dressing and secure the tube for exposure when needed for feedings, tape the dressing and tube as needed.
   f. Discard used articles according to universal precautions.

8. Maintain a semi to high-Fowler's position for 45-60 minutes following the feeding

❧ PROBLEM-SOLVING ACTIONS

1. Continuous as well as intermittent feedings can be administered with gastrostomy tube or button in place.

2. Add more formula to the syringe or container before it empties to prevent the instillation of air, tilt the container during flow to allow the air to escape.

3. Allow 10 to 20 minutes for a feeding.

4. Adjust the flow by raising or lowering the container of formula.

5. Include in I&O if being monitored.

6. Administer smaller amounts more frequently if resident complains of fullness.

7. Skin protectors such as zinc oxide or those used for urinary or bowel diversion can be used to preserve skin integrity.

8. Encourage self-feedings when possible and assist only when necessary.

❧ EVALUATION

Intermittent feedings administered via a gastrostomy safely with adequate nutritional status maintained, skin and stoma free of irritation or breakdown.

NASOGASTRIC TUBE MANAGEMENT

Anasogastric tube is a tube inserted into the stomach through the nose or mouth for the purpose of short-term enteral feedings. It is also used to aspirate gastric contents for testing. Enteral feedings (gavage) are administered if the resident is unable to digest foods through the mouth because of neurological deficits or a decreased state of consciousness that affects the ability to chew or swallow. The feedings consist of a liquid formula that is nutritionally adequate and is prepared either commercially or in food blender. They vary in constituents, concentrations, and viscosity. The amount administered daily depends on individual nutritional and fluid needs and health status. Continuous enteral feedings can be administered by gravity or infusion pump usually at a rate of 75 ml over one hour depending on tolerance. Nasogastric tube management includes the insertion, irrigation, and removal of the tube, preparation of the formula, intermittent feeding by gravity, feeding with the use of the enteral pump, and facial skin and nasal mucous membrane care. Clean technique is utilized for nasogastric tube management procedures.

❧ ASSESSMENT

Type and amount of feedings, method of administration, general nutritional and health status, adaptation to the tube feedings, condition of skin and mucous membranes for redness, crusts, irritation, tube patency and placement in the stomach

❧ NURSING DIAGNOSES

High Risk for Impaired Tissue Integrity; Self-Care Deficit, Feeding; High Risk for Aspiration; Body Image Disturbance; High Risk for Injury

❧ GOALS

Maintenance of nutritional status via nasogastric feedings without complications

❧ INTERVENTIONS

Equipment/Supplies

- Nasogastric tube with clamp
- Lubricating jelly
- Disposable gloves
- Water in a glass and straw

- Irrigation syringe and solution
- Flashlight, tongue blade

- Stethoscope

- Emesis basin and tissues
- Adhesive tape
- Wash cloth and small towel
- Formula in a measured container and water to clear the tube
- Feeding set-up with funnel or syringe barrel
- Feeding set-up with tubing, connector, pole, and enteral infusion device
- Protective ointment for skin and nares

Resident

- Explain the purpose of the procedure and expected results
- Place in semi to high-Fowler's position

❧ PROCEDURE

1. Perform handwashing.

2. Become familiar with type and size of tube, route (nasal or oral), amount and frequency of feedings, method of administration of feedings, food intolerances, or disorders that require special formula.

3. Assemble the equipment needed for procedures to be performed on a clean area within reach.

4. Perform nasogastric tube insertion:
   a. Put on gloves.
   b. Place a small towel over the chest and under the chin.
   c. Place a soft rubber tube in ice water, a firm plastic tube in warm water.
   d. Give a glass of water with a straw and a tissue to the resident to hold.
   e. Measure the distance of the tube to be inserted by placing the tip at the nose to the earlobe to the xiphoid process for nasogastric and from the lips to the earlobe to the xiphoid process for orogastric insertion.
   f. Lubricate the end of the tube, and with the tube coiled around the hand, request the resident to slightly hyperextend neck and insert the tip into the nostril or on the center of the tongue.
   g. Continue to insert through the nose downward and toward the ear while rotating the tube until it reaches the pharynx or through the mouth between the left cheek and teeth while the resident sucks on the straw.
   h. Stop at the pharynx and allow to rest, proceed with the insertion while the resident takes a sip of water and swallows, insert with each swallow until the marked distance on the tube reaches the tip of the nose.
   i. If willing, allow the resident to advance the tube while sipping water.
   j. Check the pharynx with a tongue blade and flashlight if gagging does not cease to note if tubing has coiled up in back of the mouth.
   k. Check placement by aspirating stomach contents, advance the tube farther or turn on left side and aspirate again if no aspiration; placement can also be checked by injecting air and listening to the lung sounds for swooshing indicating that the tube is in the lungs.
   l. Tape the tube in place to secure by cutting 2 inches from the end, placing the uncut end on the nose and wrapping the cut ends around the tube in opposite directions.
   m. Irrigate the tube with water to maintain patency of tube and following the feedings.
   n. Clamp tubing and pin or secure to clothing.

5. Perform nasogastric tube removal:
   a. Put on gloves and position as for insertion.
   b. Place basin receptacle in a position to receive the catheter.
   c. Remove the tape from the nose and face; discontinue any feeding procedures.
   d. Request to hold the breath and grasp the tube and pull in a smooth movement until it is completely removed.
   e. Place in the basin or wrap in the small towel, wipe the face with a damp washcloth.
   f. Provide mouthwash for mouth care and tissues to blow nose.

6. Prepare the formula to be administered:
   a. Wash top of formula container and dry, open container and pour the correct amount into a calibrated container for intermittent feedings or larger container connected to set-up for continuous feedings.
   b. Cover the container and label the remaining formula to be refrigerated with the date and time.
   c. If a powdered formula is used, mix with a liquid until completely dissolved with a blender or mixer; prepare a 24-hour amount and refrigerate the unused portion with the date and time.
   d. Warm the formula to room temperature by placing in warm water or removing from refrigerator 30 minutes prior to administration.
   e. Place the container with the formula on the tray with the other supplies needed for feedings.

7. Perform intermittent feeding via gravity:
   a. Unplug or unclamp the tube and check the placement by aspiration or injecting air and listening to the stomach for sounds.
   b. Aspirate gastric contents with a 60 ml syringe and if the residual is less than 50% of last feeding, reinject aspirate and continue with the gavage procedure.
   c. Attach the asepto syringe barrel to the feeding tube and irrigate with 30 ml water to check for tube patency.
   d. Pinch tubing and pour the formula from the measured container into the barrel or funnel and raise 12

inches higher than the stomach level.
   e. Allow to flow by gravity adding more formula before the barrel empties until all the measured amount is given.
   f. Flush the tube with 30-60 ml water to clear the formula.
   g. Clamp or plug the tube end and maintain the elevated position for 45 minutes.
   h. Remove supplies, wash, rinse, dry and cover on a tray to use for the next feeding.

8. Perform continuous feedings via enteral pump:
   a. Remove feeding container and administration set from the package and connect the tubing to the bag or container.
   b. Clamp the tubing and fill the container with a measured amount of prepared formula for continuous administration.
   c. Hang the container on a pole 24 inches above the head of the resident.
   d. Allow the fluid to fill the chamber ½ full, open the clamp and remove the air from the tubing by allowing it to fill, reclamp and cover end of tubing with a cap.
   e. Unplug or uncap feeding tube and check placement and residual as outlined above for intermittent feedings.
   f. Connect the tubing to the feeding tube and regulate the rate gtts/minute with a roller clamp, add formula to container when needed for continuous administration.
   g. If enteral pump is used, position the pump on the pole below the container of formula and attached tubing.
   h. Thread the tubing through the pump around the rotor mechanism, allow the formula to prime the tubing and set the desired rate on the pump in ml/hour, cap the tubing; check the feeding tube for patency, placement, and residual as outlined above.
   i. Turn the pump on and check alarm system, turn off and connect the tubing pump to the feeding tube.
   j. Turn pump on and begin continuous feeding or an intermittent feeding until the correct volume of formula has been administered.
   k. If intermittent, disconnect the pump tubing from the feeding tube, irrigate the feeding tube with 30-60 ml water, replug or reclamp until next feeding.
   l. Discard disposable supplies, wash, rinse, and dry reusable supplies and store for next feeding.

9. Perform face skin and nasal mucosa care:
   a. Remove and change tape to another site daily if loose or wet.
   b. Clean any dry crusting from the tube and apply protective ointment to face and nares, lips if dry.
   c. Offer mouth care (mouthwash, brushing teeth) 3 times/day.
   d. Provide chewing gum, frequent sips of water, hard candies if mouth is dry.
   e. Adjust and tape tube so that it does not rest against or place pressure on the sides of the nares.

❧ PROBLEM-SOLVING ACTIONS

1. If medications are to be given via nasogastric tube during the feeding, see Medications, Nasogastric/Gastrostomy for procedure.

2. Terminate insertion of the tube if met with resistance, remove and reinsert into the opposite nares.

3. If continuous feedings are administered, change the tubing every 4 weeks.

4. Tube placement, patency, and residual should be checked every 4 hours during continuous feedings; assess for signs and symptoms of aspiration or tube dislodgement.

5. Enteral pump can be used for both intermittent and continuous feedings but requires a specific set-up for each.

6. Include aspirate, irrigation fluid, and feedings in I & O measurements.

7. Assess for feeling of fullness, nausea, heartburn, abdominal distention, following a feeding and regulate or modify feedings to eliminate these symptoms.

8. Ensure a total of 2,000-2,500 ml/day fluid intake, 1600-1800 ml for caloric intake and the remainder in water.

❧ EVALUATION

Intermittent or continuous enteral feedings administered via nasogastric tube with daily adequate nutritional intake maintained, skin and mucosa free of irritation or breakdown

TOTAL PARENTERAL NUTRITION

Total parenteral nutrition (TPN) is the intravenous infusion of specially-prepared solutions to provide essential nutrients such as amino acids, glucose, fats, vitamins, electrolytes, minerals, and trace elements. It is administered via a central vein, usually the subclavian, using an indwelling catheter inserted by the physician with placement in the superior vena cava or right atrium. It can also be administered through a right atrial catheter (RAC) inserted through an incision in the right upper chest. A large central vein is used to dilute the solutions that are highly concentrated and would damage a smaller subcutaneous vein. Nutritional support by TPN is given when subcutaneous venous infusion or oral routes are inadequate to maintain total needs for tissue growth and the additional demands brought about by an illness. Debilitating diseases such as cancer, renal or hepatic failure and gastrointestinal disorders that affect ingestion, digestion, or absorption of nutrients are illnesses that are treated with TPN. Total parenteral nutrition management includes the preparation of the solution and fat emulsion, administration via infusion pump, solution and tubing changes, and catheter site care (see Right Atrial Catheter Management). Strict sterile technique is utilized for all procedures involved in TPN administration.

❧ ASSESSMENT

Type and amount of solutions, rate of administration, general nutritional and health status and reason for TPN, catheter insertion site for redness, edema, drainage, pain, adaptation to the presence to the catheter and treatments, I & O ratio, weight changes

❧ NURSING DIAGNOSES

High Risk for Infection; High Risk for Impaired Skin Integrity; Altered Nutrition: Less Than Body Requirements; Anxiety; Ineffective Individual Coping; High Risk for Fluid Deficit; Fluid Excess

❧ GOALS

Maintenance of optimal nutritional status via TPN without complications

❧ INTERVENTIONS

Equipment/Supplies

- TPN solution and fat emulsion in bags in correct amount and containing the correct constituents
- Padded clamp

- IV set up with filter, tubing appropriate for solutions and additives to be administered
- Reagent tablets or tape for testing glucose and ketones

- Infusion pump
- Betadine and alcohol swabs, dressings, tape with sterile dressing tray or individually wrapped sterile supplies

- Sterile gloves, face masks, protective clothing

❧ PROCEDURE

1. Perform handwashing.

2. Become familiar with the type, frequency, and volume of TPN, ability to take foods orally, type of set up and any additives, adaptation to TPN catheter placement and procedures.

3. Assemble the supplies and equipment on a clean area within reach.

4. Prepare the solutions to be administered:
   a. Check the bags of solution for clarity, discoloration, precipitate if using commercially prepared solutions.
   b. Put on sterile gloves to prepare and add to the solutions to be administered.
   c. If mixing the solutions, assemble the constituents to be added, attach a tubing to the dextrose solution container, spike the amino acid bag or bottle with the same tubing and hang on the pole, open the clamp and allow all of the amino acid solution to flow into the dextrose solution container, remove the spike from the amino acid bottle and hang the mixed solution on the pole or refrigerate until ready for use.
   d. If additives are to be added, remove the tops from the dextrose and bottles of additives and spike the additives with the shorter end of the transfer set needle and insert the other end with a needle into the dextrose container, allow all the additives (one at a time) to flow into the dextrose container on the pole with the tubing clamped, refrigerate and use within 8 hours.
   e. Other substances can be added (insulin, vitamins, medications) by injection into the latex port on the container with a syringe and needle; port should be prepared with antiseptic before injection.

5. Perform TPN administration via infusion pump:
   a. Remove solutions from the refrigerator 2 hours prior to administration and allow to stand at room temperature, check the container for leaks, clarity, and date of expiration.
   b. Spike the container with the appropriate IV tubing set up, place the tubing in the pump cassette, clamp tubing and hang the container on the pole.
   c. Attach the pump to the pole and plug into an electric outlet.
   d. Connect the cassette with the IV tubing to the pump, fill the drip chamber ½ full, unclamp and prime the tubing, cap the tubing; if a filter is used, connect it to the end of the tubing before capping, turn pump on to fill the filter and off again when filled.
   e. Set the pump to the correct rate in ml/hour to infuse the correct volume over the correct period of time
   f. Prepare the site by putting on gloves and removing the dressing and tape (see Right Atrial Catheter Management for removal and dressing change at the catheter insertion site).
   g. Cleanse the cap connector on the catheter with Betadine and alcohol swabs and clamp the catheter with the special padded clamp.
   h. Remove cover from the IV tubing and connect to the catheter end and tape to secure and prevent leakage.
   i. Remove the clamp and turn pump on and infuse the solution usually at a rate that is gradually increased every 24 hours until 125 ml/hour is administered for a continuous infusion
   j. Monitor urinary glucose during the infusion, I & O for imbalance, electrolytes for imbalances in potassium, magnesium, and phosphate.
   k. If fat emulsion is administered following TPN solution, prepare in the same manner using the appropriate tubing, remove filter or connect the infusion below the filter via a Y injection site on the TPN tubing, attach a new needle to the tubing and insert into the properly prepared catheter and tape at the connection site to secure, reset pump to administer 125 ml/hour in 4-8 hours depending on the solution concentration; usually administered 1-3 times/week.
   l. To discontinue TPN infusion, reduce the flow rate gradually by ½ for 15 minutes 30 minutes before discontinuing and ½ again for the next 15 minutes, turn pump off, clamp catheter and tubing, remove the tape from the connection and disconnect, cleanse catheter tip with antiseptic and alcohol, heparinize the catheter, replace the cap, redress and secure the catheter at the site (see Right Atrial Catheter Management for site care and dressing change).

6. Perform solution/tubing change:
   a. Assemble the new administration set up and solutions for changes in continuous TPN administration
   b. Place in a supine position and put on sterile gloves and mask.
   c. Attach the new tubing to the new TPN container and prime the tubing and filter, replace the cap on the tubing.
   d. Remove the old tubing from the pump and place the new tubing in it while on the "keep open" setting.
   e. Proceed to remove the dressing and tape from the catheter site and clean the connecting sites with antiseptic and alcohol and place on a sterile gauze square.
   f. Clamp the catheter and old tubing, disconnect and insert the new tubing.
   g. Unclamp and turn on pump to correct flow rate.

   h. Tape the connections to secure, check the set up and pump for patency and rate of infusion

   i. Return to position of comfort

7. Discard and dispose of all used supplies according to universal precautions

❧ PROBLEM-SOLVING ACTIONS

1. Portable continuous TPN can be administered for ambulatory residents.

2. Assessment of vital signs, I&O, glucose and ketones should be done during the infusion, weigh daily to determine fluid and caloric changes.

3. TPN administration can be performed without an infusion device although it is strongly preferred that one be used to ensure rate and volume.

4. Dressings should be changed every 48 hours, tubing every 24-48 hours, solutions every 24 hours, regardless of infusion type or volume.

5. TPN lines should not be used for the administration of medications or blood, other IV solutions, or CVP measurement.

6. Greshong catheters do not need clamping or heparin procedures.

7. If line becomes broken or dislodged, clamp line, turn on side, administer oxygen, call physician and/or 911 and perform any other emergency procedures needed.

❧ EVALUATION

Intermittent or continuous TPN and fat emulsion infusion administered safely and in correct volumes and at a correct rate with adequate nutritional requirements supplied, absence of skin infection or sepsis, and fluid and electrolyte complications

UNIT XII

MUSCULOSKELETAL PROCEDURES

- Assistive Devices, Ambulatory

- Assistive Devices, Bed

- Hydraulic Lift

- Immobilization Devices, Casts/Traction

- Immobilization Devices, Splints/Slings/Collars/Straps

- Muscle Strengthening Exercises

- Positioning/Movement in Bed

- Positioning the Unconscious Resident

- Range of Motion, Active/Passive/Assistive

- Restraints

- Transfer, Wheelchair/Gerichair

ASSISTIVE DEVICES, AMBULATORY

Assistive devices used for ambulation include the cane, walker and crutches. These assist in the act of walking when an individual is unable to bear the body's full weight on the legs. Canes are lightweight, adjustable or properly-sized aids that have a straight or bent shaft or three or four prongs at the base, depending on the amount of support needed to maintain steadiness. Handles are curved or straight and should be sized to the same level as the hip joint. Canes are used by those who have good balance, but lower extremity weakness. Walkers are four-pointed adjustable devices with bars at the top to grasp, bars down the sides, and one open side. They are lifted or roll with each step that is taken and require good arm strength and balance if the lifted model is used. Walkers are used by those who are unable to bear full weight on a leg or are preparing to ambulate without aid or with crutches. Crutches are adjustable lightweight aids that allow for support with the arms and hands. One type is the axillary that fits under the axillae and has a hand bar and is used for short-term assistance. Another is the Lofstrand that has a cuff that encircles the forearm and a hand bar that extends from the shaft which is used for long-term assistance. Teaching and supervising the resident in using the aids properly and safely are the primary foci of the procedures.

ASSESSMENT

Muscle strength of extremities, ability to use an aid, type of aid to be used, length of time aid is needed

NURSING DIAGNOSES

High Risk for Trauma, Impaired Physical Mobility

GOALS

Optimal ambulation with the use of an assistive aid

INTERVENTIONS

Equipment/Supplies

- Cane, aluminum or wood
- Walker with attachments
- Crutches with pads, grips, rubber tips

Resident

- Explain purpose of procedure and expected results

PROCEDURE

1. Perform handwashing.
2. Measurements and instructions for the assistive aids should be initiated by the physical therapy department, if possible.
3. If the cane is used:
   a. Ensure that the cane has a rubber tip and handgrip.
   b. Adjust the cane for the handgrip to be level with the hip joint or trochanter.
   c. Instruct to hold the cane in the hand on the strongest side of the body with the tip extended out four inches from the side of the foot and bend the arm to a 30° angle.

    d. Instruct resident to advance the cane in front of the strong leg or to advance the weak leg left to a parallel position to the cane or advance the strong leg ahead of the weak leg and cane; select the best based on the strength and coordination of the legs.

    e. Encourage to hold the cane close to the body and maintain an equal stride and timing of each step.

4. If a walker is used:

    a. Ensure that the walker has rubber tips (unless equipped with wheels) and hand grips.

    b. Adjust the height of the hand bars to allow a 30° flexion of the elbows with wrists extended.

    c. Instruct resident to stand in front of the walker with the feet about 8-12 inches apart for a safe base of support with the hands gripping the hand bars.

    d. An alternative gait (4-point gait) can be taught for the reciprocal walker.

    e. If a regular walker is used, instruct to advance the walker six inches forward and step with the strongest leg followed by the weakest leg; if the strength is equal in both legs, either leg can be moved forward first.

    f. Encourage to rest periodically when tired.

5. If crutches are used:

    a. Ensure that crutches are equipped with rubber tips, axillary pads and hand grips

    b. Adjust the crutches to measure two inches from axillae to the heel of the foot and the hand bars to allow the elbow to be flexed 30° with slightly hyperextended wrists.

    c. Instruct in 2-point gait to those with good balance (see reciprocal walker above).

    d. Instruct in 3-point gait to those who can only bear full weight on one leg; advance both crutches and the non-weight bearing leg forward about 6-8 inches and then advance the weight bearing leg forward even with the crutches and other leg.

    e. Instruct in 4-point gait to those who can bear weight on both legs; move the left crutch forward about eight inches and advance right leg parallel to the left crutch, then advance the right crutch forward and the left leg parallel to the right crutch, then left crutch ahead of the left leg.

    f. Instruct in the swing through to those using the Lofstrand, advance both crutches simultaneously and swing both legs through and even with or ahead of the crutches.

    g. Encourage to take small steps when learning to use crutches, to increase the size of the steps when feeling more secure, and to avoid bearing weight on the axillae.

❧ PROBLEM SOLVING ACTIONS

1. Provide additional instruction in sitting and getting out of a chair or using the stairs with assistive aids, if needed.

2. If a physical therapist has instructed the resident, allow adequate time and reinforcement for learning correct use of aids.

3. Assess the resident for physical and psychological readiness to use a device for ambulation (see Muscle Strengthening Exercises).

4. Proper shoes enhance the stance and gait during use of a device.

5. Provide safety by standing to the side of the resident when learning to use a device in the event assistance is needed.

6. A tote bag can be attached to the walker to carry items when the hands are holding the device.

7. Platform attachments can be added to the walker to assist in holding the hand bars for those who are unable to bear weight with the hands or arms.

❧ EVALUATION

Safe ambulation with the appropriate selection of an assistive device and correct and effective gait pattern

ASSISTIVE DEVICES, BED

Assistive devices used in bed include supplemental equipment that is attached to or placed on the bed to protect the resident and assist them to move and change positions safely. The devices are optional and selected for use depending on individual needs for safety and a protection against the complications of immobility. The more common ones are siderails, bedboard, footboard, bedcradle, metal frame and trapeze. Siderails are safety devices that prevent falls from bed and can be used to grasp when changing positions or getting in and out of bed. Bedboards are sheets or slats of wood that increase mattress firmness for those with chronic back problems. Footboards are devices that prevent footdrop. Bed cradles keep the linens off the legs and feet. The metal frame and trapeze are devices that assist the resident to lift and move in bed when needed for positioning, bedpan use, and changing linens.

ASSESSMENT

Musculoskeletal, integumentary, and bedrest status, ability to move and change positions in bed, immobilization devices

NURSING DIAGNOSES

Impaired Physical Mobility, High Risk for Impaired Skin Integrity, Activity Intolerance, High Risk for Trauma

GOALS

Safe and correct use of assistive devices while in bed to accommodate movement and positioning

INTERVENTIONS

Equipment/Supplies

- Wood or plastic footboard with padding
- Wooden slats or bedboard
- Half or full length siderails
- Bed cradle
- Metal bed frame with trapeze attached

Resident

- Explain purpose of procedure and expected results

PROCEDURE

1. Perform handwashing.
2. Bedframe and trapeze should be attached to the bed by personnel from the maintenance or orthopedic department if one is available and the trapeze hung within easy and comfortable reach for the resident to use for lifting and moving in bed.
3. If bedboards are used:
   a. Transfer the resident to a chair or stretcher.
   b. Remove the mattress and linen from the bed, secure assistance if needed.
   c. Lift the mattress and place the roll of covered slats at the head of the bed, continue to lift the mattress while unrolling the slats to the foot of the bed, position the slats so that the edges do not stick out from under the mattress.

    d. If the bedboard is a sheet of wood, remove the mattress and position the board on the bed even with the edges, replace the mattress.

    e. Replace the linens and transfer the resident back into the bed.

4. If a footboard is used:

    a. Pad the footboard with a bath blanket.

    b. Loosen the top linens at the foot of the bed and position the lip of the footboard under the mattress and fill the space between the feet and board with a folded bath blanket; avoid allowing the feet to rest.

    c. If the footboard is adjustable, position and secure the footboard at both sides of the mattress, adjust to allow for the feet to rest against it.

    d. Cover the footboard with the top linens and tuck in at the foot of the bed.

5. If siderails are used:

    a. Attach half or full length siderails to both sides of the bed depending on risk of resident falling from the bed.

    b. Pad the siderails with bath blankets if there is a risk for trauma during movements in bed.

6. If bed cradle is used:

    a. Loosen the linens at the foot of the bed and fold to expose legs and feet.

    b. Place the arm on one side under the mattress, place the arch portion over the bed and the other arm under the mattress on the opposite side of the bed.

    c. Adjust the tension attachments at the edges of both sides of the mattress.

    d. Cover the bed cradle with the top linens and tuck in at the bottom of the mattress.

❧ PROBLEM-SOLVING ACTIONS

1. Avoid tying restraints to siderails.

2. Position the footboard and bed cradle when the resident is in bed to ensure proper placement, remove when changing the bed or performing care.

3. Allow enough of the linens at the top of the bed to cover the resident adequately when a footboard or bed cradle is in place.

❧ EVALUATION

Appropriate selection and correct application/attachment of the assistive device

HYDRAULIC LIFT

The hydraulic lift is a mechanical device used to transfer a resident from and to the bed and chair. It is reserved for those who are paralyzed, obese or too weak to transfer without complete assistance. It can require two or three staff members to safely operate and accomplish the transfer.

✍ ASSESSMENT

Risk for injury to resident or staff member if conventional transfer techniques used

✍ NURSING DIAGNOSES

High Risk for Trauma; Impaired Physical Mobility; Anxiety

✍ GOALS

Safe transfer of resident to bed or chair via a mechanical lift device, correct operation of the lift

✍ INTERVENTIONS

Equipment/Supplies

- Hydraulic lift device with the sling and chains
- Wheelchair or gerichair
- Bath blanket

Resident

- Explain purpose of procedure and expected results
- Position in center of bed

✍ PROCEDURE

1. Perform handwashing.
2. Involve as many staff members as needed to ensure feeling of security by the resident, especially for the first few times the lift is used.
3. With the siderail on the far side up and the siderail on the working side down, turn the resident on the side facing you, raise the siderail, and move to the opposite side and lower the siderail.
4. Place the sling in the proper position under the buttocks with the lower edge between mid-thigh and knee, fold against the back and gently assist to turn to supine position.
5. Raise the siderail, move back to the original side, lower the siderail and pull the sling through; smooth the sling and check that the resident is centered on it.
6. Place the chair next to the head of the bed with the front facing the foot, arrange the furniture in the room to accommodate the lift.
7. Raise the bed to accommodate the lift under the bed.
8. Prepare the lift by setting the adjustable base to its widest position and lock it in place.
9. Move the lift arm to a position perpendicular to the bed and over the resident.
10. Connect the shortest strap to the shoulder portion and the longer straps to the hip portion if a 1-pieced sling is used; if a 2-piece sling is used, attach the chain to the seat portion and hook the back portion to the first, second, or third link of the chain to form a seat with two straps.

11. Check to be sure that the hooks with open ends are turned away from the resident to prevent injury and possible slipping of the hooks during the transfer.

12. Pump the lift while holding the steering arm until a sitting position is assumed and the buttocks are lifted off the bed; reassure the resident at this time.

13. Move the lift away from the bed while holding the knees with one hand to guide the movement of the resident in the sling and steadily into the chair until the proper position has been achieved (extra staff can be used for this part of the procedure).

14. While the nurse is raising and lowering the lift, one staff member can guide the resident to the chair and another can steady the chair to receive the resident.

15. Remove the straps or chains and leave the sling in place, move the lift away from the resident

16. To return the resident to bed, reverse the procedure.

❧ PROBLEM-SOLVING ACTIONS

1. Avoid any sudden movement, raising, or lowering that can frighten resident.

2. Protect the resident from harm caused by improper placement of the boom or swivel bar, hooks that are not turned away from the resident.

3. The base on the lift should be narrowed for easier storage.

4. It can allay resident anxiety if the procedure is explained step-by-step as it is being performed.

5. Avoid using the lift if oil or hydraulic fluid is noted on the floor.

❧ EVALUATION

Demonstration of safe and correct transfer of resident to bed or chair via the hydraulic lift

IMMOBILIZATION DEVICES, CASTS/TRACTION

Immobilization devices are casts and traction that are applied to restrict movement and provide the rest and support needed for healing, usually after the fracture of an extremity. Traction can also be applied to relieve pressure on spinal nerves. Casts can be made of plastic, fiberglass, or plaster of paris and are molded to the contour of the body part to be immobilized. Care involves the maintenance of the cast integrity and prevention of complications such as neurovascular or skin impairment. Traction is used to obtain a pulling force on a part of the body, such as the spine or long bones of the extremities. Care involves maintenance of the proper weight, connections and ropes.

The focus of this procedure is the management of casts of the arm or leg and the management of skin traction that is temporary and noncontinuous applied to a leg (Buck's extension) or lumbar spine (pelvic traction).

❧ ASSESSMENT

Type of injury and body part immobilized, method used for immobilization (cast, traction), pain, edema, neurovascular and skin integrity status, vital signs

❧ NURSING DIAGNOSES

High Risk for Impaired Skin Integrity; High Risk for Peripheral Neurovascular Dysfunction; Pain; Anxiety; Self-Esteem Disturbance

❧ GOALS

Safe, effective management of cast or traction application without physical or psychological complications

❧ INTERVENTIONS

Equipment/Supplies

- Traction frame on the bed
- Pillows
- Device to immobilize the leg with spreader bar, ropes, pulleys, and weights connected

- Padding, adhesive tape for cast edges
- Sandbags
- Pelvic girdle of correct size

Resident

- Explain purpose of procedure and expected results

❧ PROCEDURE

1. Perform handwashing.
2. Have the bed equipped with ropes, pulley, and correct weights.

3. If Buck's extension traction is applied:
   a. Place injured leg in proper alignment into the immobilization device equipped with a spreader bar below the foot.
   b. Place a pillow under the leg to prevent pressure on the foot.
   c. Attach weights to the spreader via ropes and pulley.
   d. Monitor traction for weights hanging freely, linens not touching traction parts, spreader not touching end of bed, ropes free of knots and in correct position, and all connections tight.
   e. Assess alignment of limb every 2 hours, numbness or pain, skin color, edema, peripheral pulse.

4. If pelvic traction is applied:
   a. Place pelvic girdle under the resident in proper position on the lower trunk so that the upper part of the appliance will fit under the umbilicus and bring the sides to the front and secure snugly with velcro or buckles.
   b. Situate so that the straps extending to the weights are straight and attach them to the ropes and spreader bar, and then to the ropes holding the weights below the pulley.
   c. Add the correct amount of weights to the hooks at the bottom of the bed; support the rope when adding weights.
   d. Check for proper body alignment and make sure the linens are not covering the device.
   e. Assess for time on and off traction, relief of pain, and any skin irritation under the appliance.

5. If cast is applied:
   a. If the cast is new, determine if dry and handle as little as possible using the palms of the hands for the first 24 hours and elevate on a pillow to reduce edema by facilitating venous return.
   b. Assess extremity digits for circulatory changes, skin color, temperature, edema, sensation and movement, peripheral pulses, redness and irritation around cast edges.
   c. Petal the cast edges with tape to protect skin or pad under edges if this does not create more pressure.
   d. Cover cast with plastic when bathing and prevent small objects from falling into the cast.

PROBLEM-SOLVING ACTIONS

1. Always explain all activities during care of cast or traction to allay the anxiety produced by these procedures.
2. Use bed protective pads when practical to protect clothing and linens.
3. Maintain all body parts in proper alignment during these treatments.
4. Inform the resident of which activities are permitted and which are to be avoided, especially as related to movement.
5. Avoid quick movements of the injured part and apply traction weights slowly and evenly.

EVALUATION

Cast or traction applied, monitored, and maintained with no skin or neurovascular complications

IMMOBILIZATION DEVICES, SPLINTS/SLINGS/COLLARS/STRAPS

*I**mmobilization devices are splints, slings, cervical collars and clavicle straps that are applied to restrict movement, support and preserve the integrity of an injured arm, shoulder or neck. Splints are rigid devices that can be used to treat a bone fracture, dislocation, or to prevent further damage of bones, joints and muscles following injury or during acute phases of chronic diseases such as arthritis. Splints are also used to treat contractures. Slings are soft, cloth devices used to immobilize an upper extremity following injury such as fracture or sprain and to help support a casted arm. Cervical collars are soft or rigid devices used to support the neck to prevent further damage to the cervical spinal cord, relieve pain, promote healing following an injury, and to treat chronic conditions such as cervical arthritis. Clavicle straps are soft cloth devices used to support the shoulders in position during the healing of a clavicle fracture.*

Devices are commercially available or can be made from cloth. Major considerations involved in administering these applications are proper alignment and optimal peripheral neurovascular function of the body part immobilized.

❧ ASSESSMENT

Type of device and reason for use (fracture, trauma, chronic disease), body part immobilized, pain, edema of body part, skin condition at site of application

❧ NURSING DIAGNOSES

Pain; Chronic Pain, High Risk for Impaired Skin Integrity; High Risk for Disuse Syndrome, High Risk for Injury; High Risk for Peripheral Neurovascular Dysfunction

❧ GOALS

Correct, safe and effective application of supportive immobilization device

❧ INTERVENTIONS

Equipment/Supplies

- Splint, sling, collar, strap as needed
- Padding
- Safety pins or other closures (tape)
- Talcum powder
- Elastic bandage, 4"

Resident

- Explain purpose of procedure and expected results
- Place in a comfortable position with body part exposed and proper alignment

❧ PROCEDURE

1. Perform handwashing.

2. If using a commercial device, instructions for application that accompany the product should be followed.

3. If a splint is applied:
   a. Select a splint that will fit the body part and immobilize the joint above or below the fracture or injury;

if used for arthritis, it should fit around the inflamed joint.
- b. Pad the splint, if needed; position and adjust with the body part in alignment.
- c. Secure with velcro, strips of cloth and pins, or tape with firmness but without compromising circulation
- d. Remove the splint periodically to assess skin and maintain cleanliness and dryness under the splint.

4. If a sling is applied:
   - a. If a commercial sling is used, unfold while supporting the extremity with the nondominant hand and guide the sling over the extremity so elbow is in the corner of the sling and fingers are exposed; place the straps over the head and adjust so fingers are slightly higher than the elbow.
   - b. If a triangular sling is used, place one end of the triangle over the shoulder of the unaffected side with the point under the elbow of the affected side while it is in about 90° flexion, bring the other end of the triangle up to the shoulder and over the affected extremity, tie ends at the side of the neck with the fingers elevated slightly higher than the elbow; secure the sling at the elbow with a safety pin or tape.

5. If a cervical collar is applied:
   - a. Position with head straight and facing forward with chin slightly elevated.
   - b. Place the collar on the neck in the proper position and fit around the neck securely.
   - c. Fasten securely in the back with velcro.
   - d. Assess neurovascular status and breathing ease to ensure that the collar is snug and supportive but not too tight.

6. If a clavicle strap is applied:
   - a. Place in a sitting or standing position with back erect.
   - b. Lightly apply talcum powder to the shoulders and axillae to prevent irritation of the skin by the strap.
   - c. If a commercial strap is used, place the strap on the resident with the apex at the back between the scapulae and place the straps over the shoulders with each strap under one axilla and through the loop, adjust the straps for proper positioning and support of the shoulders and secure with velcro.
   - d. If an elastic bandage is used, place the bandage at the center of the back in a diagonal position from the right shoulder to the left axilla, bring the lower end of the bandage under the left axilla and over the left shoulder, loop the other end of the bandage over the right shoulder and under the right axilla, secure at the back where the two ends meet, after the shoulders are in proper position.
   - e. Assess neurovascular status and skin integrity under the straps during the time worn and when removed.

❧ PROBLEM-SOLVING ACTIONS

1. All immobilization devices should be removed periodically unless a clavicle strap is used.

2. Neurovascular assessment should be performed before and during the application of any immoblization device.

3. Skin integrity should be assessed periodically when the device is removed.

4. Modifications can be made to provide immobilization, such as newspapers or magazines for a temporary splint or alternatives to commercial products such as the cloth triangular bandage or elastic bandage.

5. Use padding to protect body parts in long-term use of any immobilization device.

6. Cloth devices can be washed when soiled and, if continuous use is needed, an extra one can be kept on hand for application.

7. Gradual discontinuation of the use of a device is preferred over abrupt cessation to allow for gradual muscle strengthening.

❧ EVALUATION

Immobility device applied correctly and safely; baseline neurovascular and skin integrity status maintained

MUSCLE-STRENGTHENING EXERCISES

Exercises to strengthen muscles and develop endurance are performed to prepare a resident for ambulation with or without the use of assistive devices. These exercises condition and strengthen the muscles, especially the arms, shoulders, wrists, and hands, prior to using assistive devices. Isometric, or resistive exercises, involve pushing against a stationary object (resistive), or the contraction of a group of muscles and holding the contraction for at least 10 seconds (isometric). Usually the quadriceps, abdominals and gluteals are strengthened for ambulation and arms and shoulders are prepared for using assistive devices. Teaching and supervising the resident in practicing the exercises properly and safely are the primary foci of the procedures.

ASSESSMENT

Reason for exercises, use of assistive devices, bedrest status, physical mobility

NURSING DIAGNOSES

Activity Intolerance, Fatigue, Impaired Physical Mobility, High Risk for Trauma

GOALS

Improved muscle strength and endurance

INTERVENTIONS

Equipment/Supplies

- Rope attached to the foot of the bed
- Chair

Resident

- Explain purpose of procedure and expected results

PROCEDURE

1. Perform handwashing.
2. For resistive exercises
   a. Using a rope attached to the foot of the bed, pull body up to a sitting position to exercise arms and shoulders.
   b. While in a prone position, place the palms of the hands flat against the mattress at the shoulder level and push the upper part of the body up from the bed to exercise the arms.
   c. While sitting in a chair or in bed, place the hands on the seat or mattress and lift the hips off the chair or bed to exercise the arms.
   d. Bend the knees and push against the bed or footboard with the feet to exercise the legs.
   e. Perform each exercise at least three times, two or three times/day and increase to 10 times for each exercise as tolerated.
3. For isometric exercises:
   a. Contract the quadriceps and hold for 10 seconds and relax; repeat gradually up to ten times, two or three times/day.
   b. Contract gluteal muscles and hold for 10 seconds and relax; repeat as above.
   c. Contract abdominals and hold for 10 seconds and relax; repeat as above.

    d. Instruct to perform isometric exercises during exhalation and not to hold breath.

PROBLEM-SOLVING ACTIONS

1. Do not teach residents with cardiovascular conditions isometric exercises.
2. Range-of-motion exercises can supplement isometric exercises to increase strength and endurance.
3. The relaxation phase of the exercises is important to prevent fatigue.
4. The maximum number of exercises and frequency should be related to age, physical condition, and medical diagnoses.

EVALUATION

Demonstration of muscle strengthening exercises correctly and safely with gradual increases in strength and endurance

POSITIONING/MOVEMENT IN BED

Positioning and movement in bed involves the assistance given to change body positions for those who are unable to move independently because they are too weak or debilitated, have pain on movement, or have reduced sensorimotor function. Position changes are performed for those on temporary or permanent bedrest that require restrictions in movement. Scheduled position changes promote comfort, maintain skin integrity, prevent contractures and fatigue as well as minimize the consequences of immobility on all body systems. Supportive devices provide stabilization and protection in preventing pressure on the skin and body tissues (see Decubitus Ulcer Management). Included are low/semi/high Fowler's that include orthopneic modifications, supine, prone, lithotomy, and lateral positions, and movement to the side and up or down in bed. The Fowler's positions are used for rest and relaxation and to decrease cardiac work load and improve breathing by decreasing the pressure of the abdominal organs on the heart and diaphragm. The supine position is lying on the back and the most common position used to provide care and perform treatments. The prone position is lying on the abdomen and, although is not common, is used when posterior areas have or are at risk for pressure sores. The lithotomy position is lying in a supine position with the knees flexed, and this position is used to provide exposure to the perineal area for care and treatment procedures. The lateral position is lying on a side and is used as an alternative to enhance comfort, ease of breathing, and to prevent pressure on body parts.

The techniques involved in turning, positioning, and moving residents in bed require the nurse to use correct body mechanics to prevent back injury. Correct and supportive body alignment in positioning that maintains the joints in a neutral or in slight flexion is essential for the resident to prevent pressure on joints and muscles and to promote comfort and relaxation.

❧ ASSESSMENT

Type and frequency of position changes, ability to move in bed, joint flexibility, deformities or disabilities, supportive aids needed, skin condition at pressure points and protective aids needed, number of people needed to position resident

❧ NURSING DIAGNOSES

High Risk for Impaired Skin Integrity; Impaired Physical Mobility; Chronic Pain; Activity Intolerance; Fatigue; Ineffective Breathing Pattern

❧ GOALS

Correct and supportive positioning provided and maintained; optimal level of comfort and safety in movement and positioning

❧ INTERVENTIONS

Equipment/Supplies

- Pillows, large and small
- Sandbags
- Footboard
- Trochanter and hand rolls
- Protective devices to prevent pressure (see Decubitus Ulcer Management)

Resident

- Explain purpose of procedure and expected results
- Cover with bath blanket to provide privacy as needed

PROCEDURE

1. Perform handwashing.
2. Obtain assistance needed based on assessment of resident's ability to move in bed and type of positioning required.
3. Assemble any supportive aids needed to ensure proper body alignment, protective aids to ensure minimal pressure on skin and body tissues.
4. Place the footboard at the lower end of the mattress to relieve the pressure of the cover linens on the feet and prevent plantar flexion caused by linens that are too tight.
5. For moving a resident up in bed:
   a. Position yourself at the side of the resident with the bed at working level and remove the pillow from under the head.
   b. Position one of the resident's arms on the abdomen and the hand of the other arm on the siderail opposite of where the nurse is standing.
   c. Assuming a stance that is compliant with proper body mechanics, place one arm and hand under the buttocks and the other arm and hand under the shoulders (if two people are needed, the other person stands on the other side and places the arms and hands in the same positions while both of the resident's arms rest on the abdomen).
   d. Request the resident to flex the knees and push downwards with the feet as the nurse lifts and pulls the resident upward.
   e. Position so that the knees are in line with the knee break in the bed and replace the pillow under the head.
   f. To move a resident down in bed, follow the same procedure and lift downward without flexing the resident's knees.
6. For the supine position:
   a. After moving the resident up in bed (if needed) position the head, neck and spine in a straight line, with arms, hips, knees, and feet straight and parallel with the toes pointing upward
   b. Place a firm pillow under the head, a small pillow or pad under the ankles to raise the heels off the bed; apply cradle boots if needed to reduce pressure on the heels.
   c. Place a trochanter roll (commercial or improvised) against each hip and thigh area to prevent external rotation.
   d. Place a small pillow under each upper arm, flex each elbow slightly.
   e. Position the wrists with the fingers slightly flexed and hand rolls in place (commercial or improvised).
7. For the Fowler's positions:
   a. With the resident in supine position, raise the head of the bed 30° and raise the knee slightly or provide slight knee flexion with small pillows for low-Fowler's position.
   b. With the resident in supine position, raise the head of the bed 40-50° and raise the knee rest 10° to provide knee flexion and prevent the resident from sliding down in bed for semi-Fowler's position; place pillows under the arms with fingers over the edge as an additional comfort measure and to promote rest.
   c. With the resident in supine position, raise the head of the bed 90° and raise the knee rest to provide knee flexion for high Fowler's position; this height is also known as orthopneic position when an overbed table with a pillow is positioned over the bed for the resident to rest the head and arms to facilitate breathing.
8. For the lithotomy position:
   a. With the resident in supine position, flex and abduct the knees and hips.
   b. Place the feet flat on the bed.
   c. Drape with a bath blanket prior to care or treatment.

9. For moving a resident to the side of the bed:
   a. Position yourself at the side of the bed raised to working level.
   b. With the resident in supine position and assuming a stance in compliance with proper body mechanics, place the resident's arms on the abdomen and your hands and arms under the resident; move in segments, head and thorax first, abdomen and hips next, and legs last until positioned at the side of the bed.
   c. If two people are moving the resident, one can place the hands and arms under the upper body and the other person under the lower body and lift to the side with simultaneous movements.
   d. Continue from this position to turn to the prone or lateral positions.

10. For the prone position:
    a. With the resident in supine position at the side of the bed, place the near leg over the far leg and arms extended and placed against the body or the near arm extended in a position to reach for the siderail on the other side.
    b. Move to the far side and position the resident on the side and support the back with a pillow if two people are moving the resident, one can support the resident on the side instead of using a pillow.
    c. Move back to the near side and hold the shoulder and hip while the resident turns slowly onto the abdomen.
    d. Position the head to the side with arm raised.
    e. Place a small pillow or pad under the abdomen, shoulders knees and ankles, and allow the feet to hang over the lower end of the mattress.
    f. Place the arms prone and extended next to the body, both arms laterally from the shoulder with elbows bent and forearms parallel to the face or one arm in this position and the other forearm parallel to the body.

11. For the lateral position:
    a. With the resident in the supine position after being moved to the side of the bed opposite the direction the resident is to face, cross the far leg over the near leg and place the far arm on the abdomen and near arm in slight abduction.
    b. While facing the resident, grasp the shoulder and hip and turn on side.
    c. Place head on a pillow and pull lower shoulder and hip slightly forward.
    d. Support the back with a pillow tucked along the back lengthwise and roll it under to fit snugly.
    e. Position the bottom leg straight or in slight flexion at the hip and knee and the top leg in flexion and brought forward to rest on a pillow.
    f. Position the bottom arm in flexion and place the hand under or beside the pillow and the top arm over a pillow at shoulder level.
    g. To return to the supine position, remove the pillows and, while grasping the shoulder and hip, allow the body to return slowly to a flat position; move to the center of the bed using the same procedure as moving to the side of the bed.

✎ PROBLEM-SOLVING ACTIONS

1. Use as many small and large pillows as needed to support positions, substitute sandbags to secure a position when practical.

2. Improvise supportive aids when possible with folded towels, small pads, and commercially available sponge rubber devices to maintain alignment and protect skin from pressure.

3. Loosen restraints when positioning or moving a resident in bed.

4. Change position at least every 2 hours if resident is unable to move in bed without assistance, base frequency decisions on the resident's age, size, weight, circulatory and integumentary status and medical diagnosis.

5. Assess skin (especially bony prominences) circulatory and neurologic changes during each position change.

6. Perform range of motion exercises at each position change to prevent joint contracture and loss of muscle tone.

7. A lift sheet can be used for residents who are unable to move in bed, a plastic sheet under the lift sheet reduces friction between the sheet and bed linens.

8. Always pull when moving a resident in bed; never push as this causes more compression on the joints and tissues.

9. Sheets should be smoothed and tightened to prevent creases when positions are changed.

10. The feet should never be forced against the footboard; they can be placed against the board at a 90° angle to prevent foot drop or other devices such as a high top tennis shoe can be used.

11. The Fowler's positions may or may not include knee flexion by raising the knee gatch; knee flexion can also be achieved with a small pillow or towels.

12. Note that high-Fowler's position increases pressure on the coccyx and increases the risk of skin breakdown.

❧ EVALUATION

Safe positioning and movement in bed in correct body alignment using correct body mechanics, skin integrity, and joint and muscle mobility maintained

POSITIONING THE UNCONSCIOUS RESIDENT

The positioning and repositioning of the unconscious patient includes the same positioning procedures as performed for the conscious resident (see Positioning/Movement in Bed), the one exception is that a turning or lift sheet is used.

❧ ASSESSMENT

Level of consciousness, type and frequency of position change needed, supportive aids needed, condition of the skin at bony prominences, number of people needed to move resident

❧ NURSING DIAGNOSES

High Risk for Impaired Skin Integrity; High Risk for Injury; Sensory/Perceptual Alterations (Tactile)

❧ GOALS

Correct and supportive moving, turning, and positioning in bed using a lift sheet

❧ INTERVENTIONS

Equipment/Supplies

- Lift sheet
- Pillows of varying sizes
- Sandbags
- Footboard

- Trochanter and hand rolls
- Towels or bath blanket to fold for pads
- Protective devices to prevent pressure (see Decubitus Ulcer Management)

Resident

- Explain procedure to resident, if appropriate

❧ PROCEDURE

1. Perform handwashing.
2. Become familiar with condition of skin, type and frequency of position changes.
3. Obtain assistance depending upon movement required and weight of the resident.
4. Position the lift sheet under the resident to extend from the shoulders to below the hips.
5. Always roll the edges of the lift sheet toward the resident.
6. Maintain a broad base of support and proper body mechanics when lifting and moving the resident.
7. Place the arms of the resident across the chest and remove the pillow from under the head before moving; position the head of the bed flat if tolerated by resident.
8. Move up in bed with a nurse on each side holding the lift sheet near the shoulder and hip and, on signal, pull and lift the sheet and resident upward in the bed.
9. Pull to the side of the bed with a nurse holding the lift sheet at the shoulder and another nurse at the hips on the same side, and on signal, pull the sheet toward the nurses.

10. Turn to a side or lateral position by first pulling to the side of the bed and then grasping the lift sheet at the shoulder while another nurse grasps it at the hips and pulling the side of the sheet closest to the edge toward the nurses until the resident is on his or her side.

11. Utilize and place the pillows and other supportive devices for each position (see Positioning/Movement in Bed).

❧ PROBLEM-SOLVING ACTIONS

1. Change position as frequently as possible, at least every 2 hours.

2. Assess skin changes with each position change.

3. Use as many supportive aids as needed to maintain and secure body alignment.

4. In cases where a third nurse is needed, he/she should be situated on the opposite side of the two already positioned at the lift sheet.

5. Position pillows in the bed during the procedure to protect the resident from injury.

❧ EVALUATION

Safe movement, turning and positioning of the resident using a lift sheet and correct body mechanics, skin integrity maintained

RANGE OF MOTION, ACTIVE/PASSIVE/ASSISTIVE

Range of motion (ROM) is the extent or degree of joint movement. ROM exercises are performed to maintain joint mobility and prevent contractures. ROM is effective in maintaining muscle strength, increasing activity tolerance, and preventing complications of immobility. All residents, especially those who are immobilized or who have suffered reduced sensation or decreased level of consciousness, benefit from ROM exercises. The three types of ROM exercises are passive, active and assistive active. Each name indicates the ability of the resident to perform the exercises. Passive ROM are the movements performed by the nurse for the resident unable to do the exercises. Active ROM exercises are done by the resident without any assistance. Assistive active ROM are movements performed by both the nurse and the resident. The full ROM procedure can be a combination of exercises depending on the resident's ability and needs. Joint movements depend on the type of joint involved in the exercise. Joints are classified as pivot (cervical vertebrae 1 and 2) gliding (the other cervical vertebrae), hinge (elbow), condyloid (wrist), saddle (thumb) and ball and socket (hip).

The number of times each joint is exercised and frequency of performing the ROM exercise procedure varies with the resident's needs and tolerance. Contraindications to the procedure include joints that are inflamed or injured, as well as other conditions such as thrombophlebitis, cardiac conditions, or trauma to internal organs.

ASSESSMENT

Ability to assist, amount, type and frequency of exercises, disabilities, weakness, joint pain, paralysis, limitations of joint movement, condition of joints and muscles, and contractures.

NURSING DIAGNOSES

High Risk for Trauma; Impaired Physical Mobility; Activity Intolerance

GOALS

Correct and safe performance of ROM exercises to maintain and protect joint mobility and function

INTERVENTIONS

Equipment/Supplies

- Bath Blanket

Resident

- Explain purpose of procedure and expected results
- Place in supine position and change to lateral or sitting as needed

PROCEDURE

1. Perform handwashing.

2. Become familiar with the type and frequency of exercises, assistance needed, special considerations for specific joints.

3. Face the resident and perform the exercises with smooth and rhythmic movements, stopping if resistance is met or if the resident verbalizes pain. Support the joint and the distal extremity, holding securely above and below the joint being exercised and maintaining correct alignment of body parts during the procedure.

4. Always begin and end an exercise of an extremity in a neutral position.

5. Perform ROM exercises from head-to-toe, or whatever order is appropriate for each individual resident.

6. To perform neck exercises:
    a. Support the head with one hand and the chin with the other and move head forward with the chin toward the chest to perform flexion.
    b. Support the head with one hand on each side and move the head to the side with the ear toward the shoulder; then perform the same movement to the other side for lateral flexion.
    c. Support the head as for lateral flexion and turn the head from one side to the other to perform rotation.
    d. Remove the pillow and support the back of the head with one hand and the chin with the other hand and move the head backward to perform hyperextension.

7. To perform shoulder exercises:
    a. Position the arm in extension with the elbow straight at the side of the body with the palm facing the body and place one hand under the elbow and hold the wrist and the other hand, move the arm upward until the ear is reached to perform extension and bend the elbow for the elbow to reach above the head to perform extension-flexion.
    b. Support the arm as for extension and move the arm outward and return to the side of the body to perform abduction and adduction respectively.
    c. Support the arm as for extension and move to perform abduction, then bend the elbow to perform horizontal abduction; hold the elbow with one hand and the wrist with the other hand, and move the arm across the body until the hand touches the opposite shoulder to perform horizontal adduction.
    d. Support the arm in horizontal abduction and hold the wrist with one hand and the wrist flexed at a straight angle with the other hand, lower the forearm until the palm touches the bed and then repeat and lower the forearm until the back of the hand touches the bed to perform internal and external rotation respectively.
    e. Perform the same exercises on the opposite arm.

8. To perform elbow, forearm, wrist exercises:
    a. Support the arm as in the extension position and hold the wrist and hand with one hand and raise it at right angle to the upper arm that remains flat on the bed to perform flexion; lower the forearm to its original position to perform extension.
    b. Support the arm in extension and with one hand raise the hand while the elbow remains on the bed; place the other hand on the wrist, turn the hand with the palm up and then with the palm down to perform supination and pronation respectively.
    c. Support the arm in extension and bend the hand backward and then bend it forward to perform extension and flexion of the wrist respectively.
    d. Support the arm in extension and move the hand sideways to perform lateral flexion of the wrist and rotate the hand to perform circumduction of the wrist.
    e. Perform the same procedures on the opposite arm.

9. To perform fingers and thumb exercises:
    a. Support the arm in extension and hold the palm and wrist with one hand; straighten each finger with the other hand, then place a hand on the back of the fingers and bend them downward or take each finger individually and bend and straighten to perform extension and flexion respectively.
    b. Support the hand as for finger extension and flexion and spread each finger apart and back together again to perform abduction and adduction of the fingers respectively.
    c. Support the hand as for extension and flexion and touch each finger with the thumb to perform opposition, rotate the thumb in a circle to perform circumduction.
    d. Perform the same exercises on the opposite hand.

10. To perform hip and knee exercises:
    a. Place the leg in extension straight with the toes in an upward position and hold under the ankle

with one hand and under the knee with the other hand; bend the knee upward toward the chest and straighten again to perform extension and flexion respectively.

   b. Support the leg as for extension and move it sideways and outward and then back again to perform abduction and adduction respectively.

   c. Support the leg in extension and hold the leg above the ankle and at the knee, roll the leg inward and then outward to perform internal and external rotation respectively.

   d. Perform the same exercises on the opposite leg.

11. To perform ankle, foot and toe exercises:

   a. Support the heel of the foot with one hand and the ball of the foot with the other hand; move the foot toward the leg and pull the heel backward; then, hold the dorsum with the hand from the ball of the foot and push the foot downward and the heel backward to perform dorsiflexion and plantar flexion respectively.

   b. Support under the ankle with one hand and hold the foot with the other hand and rotate the ankle to perform circumduction.

   c. Support the ankle and foot as for circumduction and turn the foot with the sole inward and then outward to perform inversion and eversion respectively.

   d. Support the ankle with one hand and curve the toes downward toward the sole with the other hand; then straighten to perform flexion and extension respectively.

   e. Spread each toe away from the next toe and bring each toe back together to perform abduction and adduction respectively.

   f. Perform the same exercises on the opposite foot.

❧ PROBLEM-SOLVING ACTIONS

1. Perform ROM during personal hygiene procedures when possible.

2. Encourage as much independence in exercising as possible while assisting where needed. Request cooperation when practical.

3. Avoid any twisting or excessive pulling or pushing of body parts during the procedure.

4. Reinforce exercise regimen prescribed by the physician or physical therapist.

5. Maintain a base of support when performing the exercises.

6. Holding the extremity stabilizes the joint and provides more control over the movements.

7. Provide periods of rest during the exercises to prevent fatigue in the weaker resident.

8. A possible schedule of frequency can be 3-5 times for each exercise, 2-3 times per day.

❧ EVALUATION

Demonstrates ROM exercises, joint and muscle mobility and strength promoted and maintained, absence of contractures, improved mobility and activity tolerance

RESTRAINTS

R estraints are protective devices that restrict movement if there is a risk for falls or injury. Restraints should be used with caution as they can damage the skin and cause neurovascular impairment. The resident who is restrained may become restless and angry and feel helpless and afraid. Soft restraints are made of a soft fabric that ties to secure them in place. They include vest, ankle, wrist, jacket, belt and mitt restraints. Ankle and wrist cuffs are applied to the limbs and are used to restrict or to allow minimal movement of an extremity when treatments are administered. They are also used to prevent removal of IV tubing. Jacket, vest and belt restraints are applied to the chest and waist to secure an individual in a chair or bed. They should be applied so that respiratory effort is not restricted. Mitts are applied to the hands and secured at the wrist to prevent pulling at tubes, bandages and skin. They can be used with wrist restraints to further restrict arm movement. Restraints are applied and monitored according to agency policy and require careful assessment and protective interventions for the resident. The inappropriate use of or failure to use restraints have legal implications for the nurse and the agency.

ASSESSMENT

Cooperation and compliance in care, neurologic disorders, orientation and behavior changes, mental status, skin and tissues at restraint site for color, swelling, breaks, pain, pulse, numbness, type of restraint to be used

NURSING DIAGNOSES

High Risk for Impaired Skin Integrity; High Risk for Trauma; Altered Thought Process

GOALS

Safe and correct selection and application of restraint without compromising physical and psychological well being

INTERVENTIONS

Equipment/Supplies

- Restraint of appropriate size
- Protective padding

Resident

- Explain purpose of procedure and expected results

PROCEDURE

1. Perform handwashing.
2. Obtain a physician order for the restraint.
3. Assure the resident that restraint will be used only as long as necessary and can be removed as necessary.
4. If wrist or ankle restraints are applied:
   a. Wash, dry and lightly powder the skin.

   b. Place padding around the site and apply the cloth restraint over it or apply the padded side of the cuff smoothly and snugly.
   c. Fasten the cuffs by using velcro or pulling ties through the slits in the cuffs and secure with a square knot or clove hitch knot.
   d. Attach the straps to the bed frame out of reach but allowing some movement; tie with a half bow knot that can easily be untied.
   e. Slip a finger between the skin and restraint cuff to ensure that it is not too tight; check distal pulses.
   f. Apply limb restraints in patterns such as one wrist and opposite ankle, two wrists and one ankle, or both ankles and one wrist, both ankles and both wrists.

5. If hand mitts are applied:
   a. Apply the mitts over the hands.
   b. Secure at the wrists with the buckles and pull ties through the tape around the wrist and secure to the bed or chair frame.

6. If a jacket or vest restraint is applied:
   a. Place the restraint over the gown in a position that allows for turning from side to side by crossing the flaps in front and passing the tab of one flap through the slit on the opposite flap, adjust the vest for a comfortable and smooth placement on the resident.
   b. Bring the ties to the sides of the bed and tie to the frame with a bow knot.
   c. Allow enough room for ease of breathing before securing the ties.

7. If a belt restraint is applied:
   a. Place the long portion of the belt under the resident and tie the straps on each side of the bed frame.
   b. Apply the short portion of the belt around the waist and over a gown and secure with a tie or use velcro closure.
   c. Place a finger between the skin and restraints to avoid constriction.

8. Assess restraint sites every hour. Restraints should be removed for 10 minutes; exercise the joints and rotate the restraints as needed.

❧ PROBLEM-SOLVING ACTIONS

1. Always check that restraints will not tighten or pull when the bed position is changed by tying the straps to the movable part of the frame.

2. Avoid tying all restraints to one side of the bed.

3. Avoid placing buckles or knots in areas where the resident can lie on them, in areas that can be affected by pressure, over bony prominences, or where they can be reached and released or untied.

4. Maximize resident freedom when securing a restraint.

5. Follow agency policy for physician orders for restraints.

6. Restraints can be commercially made or improvised using soft cloth and roller gauze.

❧ EVALUATION

Skin and circulatory integrity maintained at restraint sites, correct and safe application and assessment of restraints, no falls from bed or chair

TRANSFER, WHEELCHAIR/GERICHAIR

ransfer *is the movement of a resident from a bed to a chair or from a chair to a bed. It also includes the movement to a sitting or standing position at the side of the bed or a standing position from a chair to a sitting position on the bed. The procedures involve various degrees of assistance depending on the strength and capabilities of the resident. Other transfer activities that are not included in this procedure are bed to stretcher/stretcher to bed and the use of a transfer board. Conditions in which assistance is usually necessary are paralysis or weakness of one or both sides. The techniques involved in transfer to and from bed and chair require that the nurse obtain extra staff to assist, if needed, and use correct body mechanics to prevent injury.*

ASSESSMENT

Muscle strength in arms, hands, legs and feet, balance when standing, ability to assist in movement in bed and to chair, age, size, mental status, presence of prosthesis, type of chair to be used

NURSING DIAGNOSES

High Risk for Trauma; Impaired Physical Mobility; Sensory/Perceptual Alterations (Tactile, Kinesthetic); Activity Intolerance

GOALS

Safe and correct transfer to and from bed and chair

INTERVENTIONS

Equipment/Supplies

- Wheelchair
- Gerichair
- Gait (transfer) belt
- Transfer (sliding) board
- Bath blanket
- Footstool

Resident

- Explain purpose of procedure and expected results

PROCEDURE

1. Perform handwashing.
2. Place the chair at a 45° angle to the bed with the seat facing the head or foot of the bed and footrests up with the uninvolved arm and/or leg nearest to the chair and lock the wheels; other placement should depend on space and IV tubes, catheters or other equipment.
3. To transfer from bed to chair:
   a. Take the pulse and blood pressure in supine position.
   b. Raise the head of the bed slowly to high-Fowler's, remove top linens, and assist to sit at the side of the bed; lower bed to position for resident's feet to rest flat and on the floor.
   c. Take pulse and note changes.
   d. Put robe and slippers on resident, and while standing in front of resident, place a hand on each

side of the chest and assist to a standing position.

    e. Support in the standing position by placing feet and knees against the resident's toes and knees, pivot toward the front of the chair and request the resident to place hands on the nurse's shoulder and pivot at the same time.

    f. Request to move back towards the chair until the legs touch it and then to grasp the arm of the chair with one hand while supporting the position with the second hand on the nurse's shoulder, flex the knees and lower the body slowly into the chair with the support of the nurse.

    g. Position in correct body alignment in the chair using pillows and pads as needed with the feet flat on the footrests and knees at a 90° angle, cover for warmth if needed.

    h. Take pulse again and note change.

4. To transfer from the chair to the bed:

    a. Position the resident in the chair at the side of the bed that allows for resident to move towards stronger and lower the bed to the correct height and lock.

    b. Assist the resident to move forward in the chair to allow one foot to be placed under the chair.

    c. While holding the resident with the hands at the waist or sides of the chest and the resident braced with the hands on each arm rest, assist to a standing position.

    d. Pivot with the resident to stand in front of the bed and, while facing the resident, assist to a sitting position on the side of the bed.

    e. Assist to remove robe and slippers and lift legs onto the bed with the back leaning against the elevated head of the bed, lower the bed slowly to a height of comfort and replace top linens.

❧ PROBLEM-SOLVING ACTIONS

1. Maintain proper positioning and body alignment to prevent pressure on bony prominence and other susceptible body tissues.

2. Obtain assistance from another staff member if resident is heavy or paralyzed; avoid allowing the resident to touch staff member's body when assisting with the transfer.

3. Provide a proper fitting chair to prevent slouching which increases the risk of pressure; modify the chair fit with the use of pillows placed at the back and sides of the client and padding to fit in space between the feet and footrests.

4. It is best to cover the chair with a bath blanket or to pad any hard-surfaced chair that might be used before seating a resident in it.

5. The wheelchair is more likely to be used when movement is desired; the gerichair when a resident remains in one place as it is stationary.

❧ EVALUATION

Safe transfer and movement to and from the bed and chair, pulse maintained within normal range during transfer

UNIT XIII

INTEGUMENTARY PROCEDURES

- Cold Applications, Dry
- Cold Applications, Wet
- Decubitus Ulcer Management
- Gelatin Compression Boot
- Hot Applications, Dry
- Hot Applications, Wet
- Stump Management
- Wound Care, Dressing Change
- Wound Care, Irrigation
- Wound Care, Suture/Staple Removal

COLD APPLICATIONS, DRY

Dry *cold applications are used to promote vasoconstriction to reduce metabolism, the movement of fluids and blood, and the movement of oxygen, nutrients and leukocytes. They are also used to remove the waste products from any area of the body being treated. Cold reduces the edema and pain associated with trauma. It reduces the conduction of sensory nerve impulses and nervous system responses to decrease muscle spasms and promote muscle relaxation. In appropriate circumstances, bleeding may be controlled by the application of cold. The most common types of dry cold application are ice bags (conduction), chemical cold packs (conduction), and reusable frozen gel packs (conduction). The optimal temperature range for cold applications is 55-65˚ F or 13-18˚ C, but this range may be modified slightly depending on the reason for the treatment, type of application, and the age of the resident.*

ASSESSMENT

Reason and type of dry cold application and expected response, area to be treated, frequency and duration, possible allergy to cold or presence of reduced sensation (tactile) to cold or reduced circulation to the area, skin condition in area of application (color, temperature, irritations or breaks)

NURSING DIAGNOSES

Pain; Impaired Physical Mobility; Altered Tissue Perfusion (Peripheral); High Risk for Impaired Tissue Integrity

GOALS

Effective and safe cold applications provided; correct monitoring of skin condition and frequency and duration of treatment, local response

INTERVENTIONS

Equipment/Supplies

- Ice bag, disposable glove
- Small towel or bag cover
- Chemical cold pack
- Frozen gel pack
- Plastic protector material or pad

Resident

- Explain purpose of procedure and expected results
- Place in position of comfort, with area to be treated exposed and properly draped

PROCEDURE

1. Perform handwashing.

2. Become familiar with type of cold application, orders for type of dry cold, times of day and duration of application; take supplies to bedside; identify resident.

3. Take temperature, blood pressure, pulse and respirations prior to application of cold treatment to serve as a comparison as temperature and blood pressure may be decreased with the vasoconstriction or may be increased suddenly as a reaction to excessive cold application.

4. If ice bag or glove is used:
   a. Fill with water and empty to check for leaks.

b. Fill bag or glove two-thirds full with ice chips.
c. Squeeze or fold bag or glove to remove excess air.
d. Place cap on bag or tie knot in glove.
e. Cover with a flannel cover or small towel and pin to secure in place.
f. Apply directly to or near part to be treated and allow to mold to body part; note time treatment began.
g. Generally apply for 20 minutes at a time, usually every 2-4 hours for 24 hours.
h. Refill container when needed and change cover if wet.
i. Note skin changes indicating potential damage, blanching, cyanosis and complaints of numbness or shivering and remove application if this occurs; check distal pulse.
j. At conclusion of the time, remove the bag or glove and dry the area with a soft cloth.
k. Empty the bag or glove of the contents, dry and store for next application.

5. If chemical cold pack is used:
    a. Select the size appropriate to the area to be treated (provides constant temperature of 50-80°F or 10-26.1°C).
    b. Activate the chemical contents according to the manufacturer's instructions by striking or squeezing the pack.
    c. Cover the pack with a small towel and pin in place.
    d. Place on area to be treated and follow *f.* through *i.* of ice bag application.
    e. At conclusion of the time, remove the pack and discard.

6. If frozen gel pack is used:
    a. Remove pack from the freezer and follow *e.* through *i.* of ice bag application.
    b. At conclusion of the time, remove the pack, disinfect and return it to the freezer for next application or future use.

✌ PROBLEM-SOLVING ACTIONS

1. Dry cold applications should be used with caution in those with circulatory impairment to prevent tissue damage.

2. Avoid chilling resident during the treatment and prolonged applications that result in shivering as the body attempts to produce heat as it shunts blood from the periphery to the internal vasculature; use blankets if needed.

3. The rebound phenomenon will occur when the maximum degree of vasoconstriction has been achieved; vasodilatation occurs if cold is continued to prevent cold damage or freezing to the tissue treated and careful timing of duration if treatment is done to avoid this (no longer than 1 hour or less than 1 hour between applications).

4. Change position or site of treatment if desired results not achieved.

5. Note presence of Raynaud's disease, arthritis, hypertension, or peripheral vascular disease prior to treatment and risks involved in cold application.

✌ EVALUATION

General condition, comfort level and safety maintained during the procedure, vital signs and skin maintained at baseline determinations, pain and edema reduced as a result of cold application

COLD APPLICATIONS, WET

Wet cold applications are used to promote vasoconstriction to reduce edema and inflammation by its effect on circulation. This inhibition of the movement of fluids and blood to the area reduces edema and pain. Wet applications also reduce bacterial activity and may be used to treat infections and to reduce body temperature by the administration of sponge baths. A wet application is considered more effective than a dry application as the moisture better facilitates conduction of the cold therapy. The most common types of wet cold applications are compresses or packs (conduction), soaks (conduction), and sponge baths (evaporation). An optimal range for cold applications is 55-85°F or 13-18°C, depending on the type used.

ASSESSMENT

Reason and type of wet cold applications and expected response, area to be treated, frequency and duration, presence of temperature elevation, possible allergy to cold or presence of reduced tactile sensation to cold or circulatory impairment, presence of wound and skin condition in area of application (color, temperature, irritations, breaks, maceration)

NURSING DIAGNOSES

Pain; Altered Tissue Perfusion (Peripheral); Hyperthermia; High Risk for Impaired Skin Integrity

GOALS

Effective and safe cold applications provided; correct monitoring of skin condition and frequency and duration of treatment, local response

INTERVENTIONS

Equipment/Supplies

- Basin of water with chipped ice
- Bath thermometer
- Ice bag, disposable glove 2/3 filled with chipped ice and covered appropriately

- Plastic protector material to cover wet treatment and linens
- Wash cloth, gauze dressing, towel or flannel material
- Large container of water and chipped ice for soak

Resident

- Explain purpose of procedure and expected results
- Place in position of comfort, with area to be treated exposed and properly draped

PROCEDURE

1. Perform handwashing.
2. Become familiar with type of cold application, times of day and duration of off and on application; take supplies to bedside and identify resident by wristband.
3. Take temperature, blood pressure, pulse, and respirations prior to treatment to serve as a comparison as changes may occur with vasoconstriction.
4. If compresses or pack is used:
   a. Measure temperature of water (optimal for compresses is 59°F or 15°C).

   b. Place gauze dressing or cloth in the water, soak and wring out.

   c. Apply the compress or pack to the area and note the time treatment began.

   d. Cover the material with the waterproof covering and secure in place with tape.

   e. Place the ice bag or glove over the area to maintain cold if appropriate; see Cold Applications, Dry for procedure to prepare ice bag or glove.

   f. If ice bag or glove is not used to maintain temperature, change the compress or pack as needed.

   g. Generally, apply for 20 minutes at a time at frequency ordered depending on the reason for the treatment.

   h. Note skin changes indicating potential damage, blanching, cyanosis, maceration, complaints of numbness, chilling.

   i. At conclusion of the time, remove the compress or pack and dry the area with a soft cloth.

   j. Discard disposable liquid and material, dry cloths and store for next application.

5. If soak is used:

   a. Take temperature of water in basin large enough to fit part to be treated.

   b. Submerge part to be treated in the water and note the time treatment began.

   c. Generally soak for 20 minutes at a time at frequency ordered; add ice to the water when needed to maintain the desired temperature.

   d. Note skin changes indicating potential damage as with the application of compresses or packs and complaints of chilling or discomfort.

   e. Remove treated part from the soak and dry with soft cloth at conclusion of therapy.

   f. Discard disposable material; dry container and store for next application.

6. If sponge bath is used:

   a. Refer to Bath, Cooling Sponge for procedure to perform this activity to lower body temperature.

❧ PROBLEM-SOLVING ACTIONS

1. Wet cold applications should be used with caution in those with circulatory impairment to prevent tissue damage.

2. Avoid chilling of resident during the treatment by providing additional warmth as needed (blankets, warm liquids to drink).

3. Note presence of possible rebound phenomenon when maximum degree of vasoconstriction has been reached causing vasodilatation to occur to prevent cold damage or freezing to the tissue treated; perform careful and accurate timing of treatment duration (no longer than 1 hour or less than 1 hour between applications).

4. Change position or site or discontinue treatment if desired results not achieved or tissue damage noted; remain with resident who is neurologically or congnitively impaired.

5. Note presence of Raynaud's disease, arthritis peripheral vascular disease, or other conditions in which cold treatments may be contraindicated and the risks involved in a cold application for these residents.

6. Adhere to principles of sterile technique if an open wound or any break in the skin is within the area of treatment and dispose of supplies according to universal procedures.

❧ EVALUATION

General condition, comfort level, and safety maintained during the procedure, vital signs and skin condition within baseline parameters, reduction of pain and edema noted

DECUBITUS ULCER MANAGEMENT

Decubitus or pressure ulcer management is the treatment of skin breakdown caused by sustained pressure of the tissue over a bony prominence resulting in ischemia as the blood supply to the area is reduced, friction and shearing that damages the skin. Other factors are aging skin, inadequate nutrition, reduced fat, loss of muscle mass, and incontinence. The most common sites for decubiti are the sacrum, iliac crests, heels, scapulae, ears, head, and elbow. Ulcer formation begins with redness and blanching and progresses to the destruction of the epidermis and dermis with treatment varying according to the stage of development. Sterile techniques are required to perform decubitus ulcer care.

ASSESSMENT

Age of resident and condition of skin, presence of conditions predisposing to or increasing stage of decubitus formation and site(s) involved, nutritional and fluid intake, size and characteristics of the pressure ulcer

NURSING DIAGNOSES

Impaired Tissue Integrity; High Risk for Impaired Skin Integrity; High Risk for Infection; Altered Tissue Perfusion (Peripheral)

GOALS

Relief of pressure and restoration and progressive healing of tissues; effective and correct prevention treatment and monitoring of pressure ulcer

INTERVENTIONS

Equipment/Supplies

- Sheepskin, eggcrate mattress
- Lotion for massage
- Ointments, sprays, pastes, powders to protect skin
- Skin barrier, transparent film, hydrocolloid, polyurethane foam membrane, hydrogel dressings
- Pillows, protective devices for heel, elbow

- Wound irrigation supplies, wound dressing and wet compress supplies
- Sterile and disposable gloves
- Basin of warm water, wash cloth, soft towel, and commercial pH neutral skin cleanser
- Medications and solutions as ordered

- Protective pads

Resident

- Explain purpose of procedure and expected results
- Place in position of comfort that allows for exposure of the area for treatment, properly drape for privacy and warmth and place protective pad in position if needed

PROCEDURE

1. Perform handwashing.

2. Become familiar with the type and extent of breakdown and orders for treatment, type and frequency of treatment, preventive measures to be used.

3. Take supplies to bedside and identify the resident by wristband.

4. Prepare a sterile field on a nearby table and open sterile packages, place on field and pour liquids if used; include sterile irrigation supplies and any special medications or debridement agent and supplies needed (see Sterile Technique for opening packages, pouring liquids, putting on gloves and see Wound Management, Dressing Change and Irrigation).

5. Put on disposable gloves and gently remove the existing dressing and discard in a waterproof bag.

6. Wash and rinse the skin around the breakdown with warm water and pH neutral or a commercial cleanser, gently pat dry and massage the area, discard gloves in waterproof bag.

7. Note, identify and measure size of ulcer and characteristics of any drainage, phase of wound healing and stage of pressure ulcer.

8. Wash hands and put on sterile gloves.

9. Apply any ointments, sprays, or pastes to protect the skin from moisture if needed, use a sponge applicator or tongue blade, direct any spray away from any open breaks.

10. Apply a dry dressing with Telfa and secure with tape or apply a transparent permeable adhesive dressing to the ulcer depending on the stage of the ulcer, usually Stages I & II.

11. Cleanse area with sponges and normal saline solution, irrigate as appropriate from the cleanest to least clean area and discard used materials in disposal bag (see Wound Care, Irrigation).

12. Apply ordered medication, debriding agent, gelatin sponge to prevent infection or absorb secretions depending upon the stage of ulcer hydrocolloid, hydrogel, polyurethane foam.

13. Remove gloves and discard in disposal bag with other used articles and according to universal precautions.

14. Store reusable supplies for next treatment.

15. If preventive care is to be given:
    a. Wash and rinse area with warm water and mild soap, pat dry and maintain dryness of any reddened area.
    b. Expose to the air; lubricate skin as needed with cornstarch.
    c. Spray benzoin to area if necessary to protect the skin or apply other protective ointments or pastes (zinc oxide or petroleum jelly).
    d. Utilize protective measures to reduce or control pressure on an area such as foam, water or air mattress on bed and foam, gel, or air seat cushions on a chair.
    e. Reposition every 2 hours or more often, depending on ability of resident to move in bed or chair using care to prevent damage to fragile skin; reduce shearing and friction potential.
    f. Assist with or perform range of motion exercises to promote circulation and prevent joint and muscle complications.
    g. Change linens and maintain smoothness and perform other measures to ensure a dry environment for skin; cleanse and dry skin after soiling.
    h. Assist to shift body weight in chair every 30 minutes to prevent pressure on a part and avoid head of bed elevation of more than 30 degrees for prolonged periods of time; a lower position nearer to prone is desirable.
    i. Ensure nutritional and fluid intake.

❧ PROBLEM-SOLVING ACTIONS

1. Shaving of the area may be necessary to prevent contamination and to allow the area to be taped with a dressing without pulling the hair.

2. Nutritional and fluid intake should include vitamin C, protein and additional calories.

3. Consult nutritionist for evaluation of dietary and fluid intake.

4. Constant vigilance for infection of a decubitus is essential.

5. Ulcer measurement should be done to determine degree of healing.

6. Avoid massage of pressure areas and use of donuts or heat lamps.

7. Prevent the linens from becoming tight which may cause pressure to the toes or other areas; avoid friction and shearing when moving in bed by pushing or pulling resident.

8. Provide trapeze to facilitate movement while in bed.

9. Combine the products available for care and dressings to provide the best results such as one to maintain moisture of wound, absorb excess exudate, and a cover that will retain moisture and provide a dressing.

❧ EVALUATION

Decubitus care performed safely without incident, progressive decrease in the size of the ulcer with absence of infection; preventive measures resulting in absence of redness of skin at pressure points or in any area

GELATIN COMPRESSION BOOT

Gelatin compression boots (Unna Boots) are medicated dressings that are applied to a foot or leg to treat a venous ulcer. They serve as a protection to the limb and exert pressure to the veins to promote healing. The material may be applied to the limb in paste form or applied by wrapping the limb with a commercially-prepared gauze that is treated with the paste. Clean technique is used to prevent any infection to the ulcerated area.

ASSESSMENT

Presence of venous ulcer, infection, presence of dermatitis resulting from impaired venous circulation, allergy to the material used from compression boot, presence of edema of the limb, condition of skin around area of ulcer

NURSING DIAGNOSES

Impaired Skin Integrity; Altered Tissue Perfusion (Peripheral); Impaired Tissue Integrity; High Risk for Infection

GOAL

Improvement in venous ulcer healing; safe and correct application and removal of gelatin compression boot

INTERVENTIONS

Equipment/Supplies

- Unna paste and roller gauze
- Commercially prepared bandage with Unna paste
- Elastic bandage
- Scissors
- Towel to place under foot or protective cover
- Disposable gloves

Resident

- Explain purpose of procedure and expected results
- Place in sitting position with leg to be treated resting on footstool with knee in slightly flexed position

PROCEDURE

1. Perform handwashing, put on gloves.
2. Become familiar with action of the paste and expected response from its use.
3. Take supplies to resident and identify him/her by wrist band or other method.
4. If paste and roller gauze is used:
   a. Spread the paste evenly on the leg and foot.
   b. Apply roller gauze over the paste.
   c. Spread another layer of paste over the gauze.
   d. Apply another layer of gauze.
   e. Repeat paste application and gauze layering a second time or as many times as needed for a firm supportive boot.
5. If commercially prepared bandage is used:
   a. Start at the foot and apply two circular turns to anchor the bandage.
   b. Continue to bandage the foot with the gauze and move up the ankle using figure eight turns until the

          area is completely covered.

   c. Continue up the leg to knee level with spiral turns and overlap the previous turn by about ½ of the bandage width.

   d. Mold the gauze to the leg firmly with even pressure and slit the boot below the knee to prevent circulation impairment as the boot sets.

   e. Apply an elastic bandage to protect clothing and linens from soiling (see Ace Elastic Bandage).

   f. Elevate leg on pillow for 30 minutes to allow for drying.

6. Note color and temperature of digits which indicated circulatory impairment (cool, purplish color, pain).

7. Remove by cutting with a scissors, assess skin and ulcer, reapply boot in a week or as ordered.

8. Discard used boot, cleanse skin with warm water and mild soap and pat dry with a soft cloth.

❧ PROBLEM-SOLVING ACTIONS

1. Allow toes to be exposed when applying the boot to allow for checking of circulation as the boot dries.

2. Avoid any damage to the boot that will affect the desired therapeutic effect.

3. Cover boot with plastic bag and secure while bathing to prevent softening.

4. Maintain smooth consistent turns when applying bandage and avoid making any reverse turns as bandaging moves up the leg.

❧ EVALUATION

Progressive healing of ulcer, leg protected from trauma and injury, absence of circulatory impairment or infection at ulcer site

HOT APPLICATIONS, DRY

Dry *heat applications are used to promote vasodilatation which increase blood flow to an area resulting in an increase in nutrients, oxygen, antibodies, and leukocytes and the removal of waste products of the metabolic process. This causes an increase in the discharge of pus and promotes tissue healing. Its use relieves pain and reduces muscle spasms that result from ischemia in conditions that prevent normal blood flow. The most common types of dry heat applications and their methods of heat transfer are hot water bags (conduction), aquathermia pads (conduction), chemical hot packs (conduction), and heat lamps (conversion). An optimal temperature range for heat applications is 105-125° F or 40.5-51.6° C depending on the reason for the treatment, type of application, and the age of the resident.*

❧ ASSESSMENT

Reason and type of dry heat application and expected response, area to be treated, frequency and duration, presence of reduced sensation (tactile) to heat or impaired circulation to the area, skin condition in area of application (color, temperature, irritation, open wound)

❧ NURSING DIAGNOSES

Pain; Impaired Physical Mobility; Altered Tissue Perfusion (Peripheral); High Risk for Impaired Skin Integrity

❧ GOALS

Effective and safe dry heat applications provided; correct application and monitoring of skin condition and local response

❧ INTERVENTIONS

Equipment/Supplies

- Hot water bag and cover
- Chemical heat pack
- Heat lamp with proper size bulb
- Measuring tape
- Bath thermometer
- Plastic protector material or pad
- Aquathermia pad and cover
- Distilled water

Resident

- Explain purpose of procedure and expected results
- Place in position of comfort, with area to be treated exposed and properly draped; protective cover in place

❧ PROCEDURE

1. Perform handwashing.
2. Become familiar with type of heat application, time of day and duration of treatment.
3. Take supplies to bedside and identify resident by wristband.
4. Take vital signs prior to the application to serve as a comparison as blood pressure may decrease with vasodilatation as blood is removed from internal organs into the circulation.
5. If hot water bag is used:
   a. Place hot water from the tap in a pitcher.
   b. Take temperature of the water with a bath thermometer (optimal temperature for an elderly resident

105-115°F or 40.6-46.1°C).

   c. Pour water into the bag that has been preheated until two-thirds full.

   d. Expel excess air by squeezing or folding bag and place cap or secure top of bag to allow bag to mold to body part and enhance conduction of heat.

   e. Dry bag and cover.

   f. Apply directly to or near part to be treated and note the time treatment began.

   g. Generally, apply for 20 minutes at a time or as ordered and assess skin for potential damage, redness, complaints of burning when application removed or changed.

   h. Refill container when needed and change cover if wet to maintain desired temperature and comfort.

   i. At the conclusion of the time, remove the bag, empty and dry, store for next treatment; allow to fill with air and cap to prevent bag from sticking.

6. If chemical heat pack is used:
   a. Select the size appropriate for the area to be treated.
   b. Activate the chemical contents according to the manufacturer's instructions by striking or squeezing the pack (provides a constant temperature of 105-115°F or 40.5-46°C).
   c. Cover the pack with a small towel and pin in place.
   d. Place on area to be treated and follow *f.* and *g.* of hot water bag application.
   e. At conclusion of the time, remove the pack and discard.

7. If aquathermia pad is used:
   a. Place cover on pad and secure in place.
   b. Fill the water reservoir two-thirds full with distilled water and place on a table slightly higher than the area to be treated to allow the flow of water through the pad by gravity.
   c. Fill the pad with the water by tilting it to eliminate any air bubbles.
   d. Plug into an electric outlet and set the thermostat to the desired temperature (optimal temperature is 105°F or 40.5°C).
   e. When desired temperature is reached, apply the pad to the area to be treated for duration and frequency (or continuous) of the application as ordered.
   f. At conclusion of the treatment, remove the pad, turn thermostat to off and empty the water reservoir and pad; dry and store for future use.

8. If heat lamp is used:
   a. Place correct-sized bulb into the lamp and plug into an electric outlet.
   b. Allow the lamp to heat.
   c. Remove any metallic objects near the treatment site or lamp and any dressing if present.
   d. Position lamp at the resident's side to prevent injury if the lamp falls.
   e. Place lamp 14-16 inches from treatment area depending on size of bulb (optimal bulb size is 40 watts)
   f. Generally apply for 10-15 minutes for first treatment to determine residents's tolerance to the heat with assessment every 5 minutes and then for 15-20 minutes for subsequent treatments.
   g. Discontinue treatment if skin becomes reddened.
   h. At conclusion of the treatment, remove the lamp, redress the area, if appropriate, and store the equipment for future use.

❧ PROBLEM-SOLVING ACTIONS

1. Dry heat applications should be used with caution in those with circulatory impairment to prevent tissue damage and in areas of scar tissue or in the presence of stomas.

2. Equipment with frayed cords or other damage should be replaced.

3. Ensure that the controls of the heating apparatus is out of the reach of the resident or instruct to refrain from changing the controls that regulate the temperature.

4. Avoid use of pins on a heating apparatus that could damage the device or cause leakage or burns.

5. If thermometer is not available, use inner aspect of arm to test temperature of device.

6. Change position or site of treatment if desired results are not achieved.

7. The rebound phenomenon will occur when the maximum degree of vasodilatation has been relieved and tissue congestion occurs; vasoconstriction then takes place and the risk of burn is present and loss of

the therapeutic effect of the heat; careful timing and duration of the treatment is done to avoid this (no longer than 30 minutes for a heat application).

8. Cold applications may be replaced with heat applications following trauma in 48 hours or after edema is no longer forming.

9. Avoid use of ointment or lotions prior to application of dry heat as they may provide an additional conductor of the heat and cause burns.

10. Avoid covering a heat lamp and area to form a tent as this increases the intensity of the heat; no flammable material should touch the bulb of a lamp or bed cradle if used; the goose neck of the lamp should not touch the residents, bed cradle or other metal.

11. Position heat source or resident to allow for change and movement away from heat if desired or needed.

❧ EVALUATION

General condition, comfort level and safety maintained during the procedure, vital signs and skin maintained at baseline determinations, pain relieved and healing improved and progressing

HOT APPLICATIONS, WET

*W*et heat applications are generally used to promote vasodilatation to increase blood flow to a small or large area resulting in an increase in nutrients, oxygen, antibodies, and leukocytes and the removal of waste products of the metabolic process. This promotes tissue healing and increases discharge of pus present in infection. It also provides relaxation of muscles by increasing nerve impulse conduction by stimulating the thermal receptors in the skin. Medications may be prescribed and added to the solution used for wet heat applications, usually in soaks or packs applied to open wounds. The most common types of wet heat applications and their methods of heat transfer are compresses or packs (conduction), soaks (conduction), hydrocollator packs (conduction), sitz or tub baths (convection). An optimal range for heat application is 90-115°F or 32-46°C depending on type of application and reason for treatment.

ASSESSMENT

Reason for and type of wet heat application and expected response, area to be treated, frequency and duration, presence of reduced sensation (tactile) to heat or impaired circulation to the area, skin condition in area of application (color, temperature, irritation, open wound)

NURSING DIAGNOSES

Pain; Altered Tissue Perfusion (Peripheral); High Risk for Impaired Skin Integrity

GOALS

Effective and safe wet heat applications provided: correct application and monitoring of skin condition and local response

INTERVENTIONS

Equipment/Supplies

- Basin and hot water
- Gauze dressings commercially prepared for sterile wet compresses
- Prescribed medication
- Dressings for wound following treatment
- Disposable gloves/sterile gloves if needed
- Tape
- Bathroom thermometer
- Large container of water for soak
- Plastic protector material or pad
- Hot water bag or aquamatic pad with necessary supplies for preparation
- Wash cloth, large towel or material
- Hydrocollator packs, towels, container of distilled water, tongs or gloves

Resident

- Explain purpose of procedure and expected results
- Place in position of comfort, with the area to be treated exposed and properly draped; protective cover in place

❧ PROCEDURE

1. Perform handwashing.
2. Become familiar with type of heat application, times of day and duration of treatment.
3. Take supplies to bedside including medication and identify resident by wristband.
4. Take vital signs prior to the application to serve as a comparison as blood pressure may decrease with vasodilation as blood is removed from internal organs to the circulation when the vessels are dilated.
5. If compress or pack is used:
   a. Place hot water from tap in a basin large enough to accommodate the size of compress or pack.
   b. Measure the temperature of the water (optimal for compresses is 105°F or 40.6°C).
   c. Add medication to the solution if ordered; if solution used is available mixed, heat the solution by placing the bottle in hot water for about 20 minutes or until desired temperature achieved.
   d. Place the gauze compress, towel or cloth in the solution or water, soak and wring out with instruments or gloved hands.
   e. After testing hot compress place directly on area to be treated and note the time treatment began (remove dressing, if appropriate, prior to application).
   f. Cover the application with waterproof material and secure in place.
   g. Apply hot water bag or aquathermia pad over the application to maintain temperature or change compresses or packs every 5-15 minutes as needed; see Heat Applications, Dry for procedure to prepare hot water bag or aquathermia pad.
   h. Generally apply for 20 minutes, depending on reason for the treatment.
   i. Note skin changes indicating potential damage, redness, maceration, complaints of numbness, pain, or burning feeling.
   j. At conclusion of the time, remove the compress or pack and dry the area with a soft cloth; redress if wound is being treated.
   k. Discard disposable liquids and material, dry cloths and store for next application.
   l. If skin is broken or open wound present, sterile technique must be used in performing the treatment and use articles disposed of according to universal precautions; packaged sterile compresses that may be heated are available for use if small area is to be treated.
6. If soak is used:
   a. Place hot water from tap or heated medicated solution in container of appropriate size.
   c. Submerge part to be treated in the solution or water and note time the treatment began (remove dressing if appropriate prior to immersion).
   d. Generally, soak for 20 minutes; add warm water to the container when needed to maintain the temperature.
   e. Note skin changes indicating potential damage, redness, pain, burning.
   f. Remove treated part from the soak and dry with soft cloth at conclusion of therapy; redress if wound being treated.
   g. Discard disposable material and fluid according to Universal Precautions, dry container and store for next application.
7. If sitz bath is used:
   a. Refer to Bath, Sitz for procedure to perform this activity to treat perineal and rectal area with heat application.
8. If warm/hot bath is used:
   a. Refer to Bath, Tub for procedure to perform this activity to promote relaxation and relieve pain.
9. If hydrocollator pack is used:
   a. Fill container with distilled water and set thermostat at desired temperature (usually 140°F or 60°C) and place packs in water.
   b. Allow 20 minutes to heat packs initially or 5 minutes to reheat packs.
   c. Prepare towel to wrap pack, possibly 3 towels or more.
   d. Remove packs from container with tongs or gloves at the corners and allow to drip over the container to remove excess water.
   e. Place packs in center of towel and fold the sides of the towel over the pack and continue one towel at a time until the desired covering is achieved.
   f. Place the wrapped pack on the area to be treated.

g. Place rolled towels at the sides to support the pack if needed or secure in place or support a joint being treated with a rolled towel.
h. Generally, apply for 20 minutes, replace with a fresh pack being heated in the container if needed.
i. Note skin condition every 5 minutes initially and then at 10 minutes intervals for redness, pain, and burning sensation.
j. At conclusion of the time, remove the packs, store pack in machine or plastic bag, launder towels.
k. Discard water from container, dry area with a soft cloth.

❧ PROBLEM-SOLVING ACTIONS

1. Wet heat applications should be used with caution in those with circulatory impairment to prevent tissue damage and in areas of extensive skin breakdown.

2. If thermometer not available, inner aspect of arm may be used to test temperature of water or solution.

3. Limit heat application to 30 minutes to prevent rebound phenomenon which will reverse therapeutic effect and may burn.

4. Heat application may replace cold following trauma if edema is no longer forming.

5. A cover may be used in soak treatment to maintain the water temperature.

6. All metal objects should be removed before heat treatment as the metal may be heated and cause a burn.

7. Wet towels should not be used for hydrocollator packs; they should be replaced with dry towels when replacing a pack.

8. Treatments should be discontinued if skin maceration, blistering is present as wet heat has a greater risk for causing burns since moisture conducts heat.

9. Adhere to principles of sterile technique if an open wound is being treated.

❧ EVALUATION

General condition, comfort level, and safety maintained during the procedure, vital signs and skin condition within baseline parameters, pain relieved and wound healing progressing as infection subsides

STUMP MANAGEMENT

S tump care is a combination of routine skin cleanliness, monitoring, muscle exercises, and routine prosthesis cleaning and adjustment to ensure proper fit. This includes the care of a healed stump of the arm or leg to prevent skin irritation or breakdown and correction of any prosthesis malfunction that may result in skin damage.

ASSESSMENT

Condition of skin at stump site, ability to comfortably use the prosthesis, psychological effect of loss of limb

NURSING DIAGNOSES

High Risk for Impaired Skin Integrity; Body Image Disturbance; Impaired Physical Mobility

GOALS

Effective and safe stump and prosthesis care provided; correct monitoring of skin and prosthesis and removal and application of prosthesis

INTERVENTIONS

Equipment/Supplies

- Basin of warm water and mild soap
- Wash cloth and soft towel
- Alcohol and sponges
- Stump cover or sock
- Lubricating oil for prosthesis

Resident

- Explain purpose of procedure and expected results
- Place stump in position of comfort with necessary support and properly draped

PROCEDURE

1. Perform handwashing.
2. Become familiar with type of prosthesis and duration of time used, when surgery was performed, ability to ambulate and perform activities of daily living (ADL).
3. Take supplies to bedside and identify resident by wristband.
4. Remove the stump sock, assess skin for irritation, redness, swelling, breaks.
5. Gently wash the stump and pat dry.
6. Apply alcohol and massage the stump to enhance firming of the tissues.
7. Perform muscle strengthening exercises to the stump as well as unaffected limbs which will enhance use of the prosthesis unaffected limb should also be exercised.
8. Apply a clean stump sock with the placement of any seams away from the incisional site or part of the stump that receives pressure when placed into the prosthesis.
9. Reapply prosthesis and secure.
10. To care for prosthesis:
    a. Cleanse the socket of the prosthesis with soap and warm water and dry well.

    b. Oil the prosthesis if allowed.

    c. Adjust, if possible, or refer malfunction or complaints about fit to a prosthetist.

    d. Clean and check shoe on the prosthesis and change if needed.

    e. Reapply the prosthesis by placing it over the stump or applying an insert over the stump and then insert this into the prosthesis.

❧ PROBLEM-SOLVING ACTIONS

1. Secure properly-sized and fitting stump socks and always have a clean one on hand for use; soiled socks may be washed and allowed to dry for reuse.

2. Avoid using any lotion products on the stump as these may be irritating and provide a medium for bacterial growth.

3. Elevate the stump for comfort and if edema is present; avoid prolonged bending of a knee to prevent contracture.

4. Cleansing of the stump need not necessarily precede application of the prosthesis but may be done at any time depending on preference and if swelling is present.

5. Avoid use of the prosthesis if skin on stump is irritated, red, or broken.

6. Store the prosthesis in a clean, safe place when not in use.

❧ EVALUATION

Skin at stump site free of redness and irritation, prosthesis properly cared for and removed and applied as appropriate

WOUND CARE, DRESSING CHANGE

Wound dressing change is the removal of soiled bandages, cleansing of a wound and the reapplication and securing of clean dry dressings or bandages. The dressings are applied to cover and protect a wound, and in some cases, to support and provide pressure to the wound when needed. They may also be used to absorb drainage and prevent drying if the wound is open. Sterile principles and technique are required to perform any type of wound care to prevent infection. Wound dressing change may be applied as a wet dressing (saline or medicated) and allowed to dry, removed and then redressed with dry bandages. This type of dressing is used to debride an open wound that must heal by granulation (see Decubitus Ulcer Care).

ASSESSMENT

Type of wound and dressing needed, time of day and frequency of dressing change, skin condition around wound (irritation, redness, swelling, rash), healing status, presence of nutritional and fluid deficiency affecting healing

NURSING DIAGNOSES

Impaired Skin Integrity; Impaired Tissue Integrity; High Risk for Infection

GOALS

Effective and safe dressing change and wound care provided; correct monitoring of skin and wound condition and healing

INTERVENTIONS

Equipment/Supplies

- Sterile dressing tray or individually wrapped sterile supplies appropriate to wound care

- Sterile gloves and disposable gloves

- Adhesive remover

- Nonallergic tape

- Extra sterile dressings (ABD, gauze squares, occlusive)

- Sterile solution (normal saline, antiseptic)

- Cotton applicators (sterile), dry or with antiseptic

- Transparent, semipermeable film adhesive dressing

Resident

- Explain purpose of procedure and expected results

- Place in position of comfort that allows exposure to the area without causing tension on the wound, properly draped for privacy and warmth

PROCEDURE

1. Perform handwashing.

2. Become familiar with the type of wound and dressing needed, frequency of dressing change, whether dressing is wet or dry and solution ordered.

3. Take supplies to the bedside and identify the resident by wristband.

4. Set up sterile field on a nearby table and open sterile packages, place on field and pour liquid in basin if used (see Sterile Technique for opening packages, pouring liquids, putting on gloves).

5. Put on disposable gloves and gently remove dressing, pull adhesive in direction of wound while stabilizing the skin; loosen dressing with normal saline if dried and stuck to the wound to prevent pulling at wound site.

6. Discard soiled dressing and tape in a waterproof disposal bag.

7. Cleanse the skin of any old adhesive tape with remover and rinse area to remove chemical from skin; remove gloves and discard in disposal bag.

8. Note skin and wound condition and characteristics of drainage if present.

9. Wash hands and put on sterile gloves.

10. Cleanse wound with an applicator or a gauze dipped into an antiseptic solution with a forceps or commercially prepared antiseptic swabs using strokes from the cleanest to most contaminated area; use one swab or applicator per stroke and start at the wound and move outward.

11. Discard used swabs or applicators in disposal bag.

12. Allow to dry and apply 4x4 gauze squares, skin protectant, ABD pad as needed or ointment if ordered to protect skin; layer the dressing evenly to extend well beyond the wound on all sides; remove gloves and discard.

13. Apply tape to secure the dressing or Montgomery straps if appropriate, especially if resident is obese.

14. Discard used supplies according to Universal Precautions.

❧ PROBLEM-SOLVING ACTIONS

1. Dressings may be reinforced if a complete change is not warranted.

2. Allergic reactions to the tape may be avoided by the use of nonallergic tape or tape made of material that does not irritate the resident's skin.

3. Gloves should be worn to protect both the resident and practitioner from transmission of microorganisms.

4. Cleansing should be done until all drainage and debris are removed from the wound

5. Dressings may be covered and taped in place in a window configuration during bathing to protect it from dampness.

6. Dressings may be cut with a sterile scissors to fit around tubes or drainage devices.

7. Wet dressing of gauze and normal saline can be applied for a limited time to keep an open wound moist and allow for tissue granulation.

❧ EVALUATION

Dressing change performed safely without incident, progressive wound healing noted with absence of infection

WOUND CARE, IRRIGATION

*W*ound irrigation is the instillation of fluid to remove drainage and debris to promote healing. Antiseptic or antibiotic solutions may be used to prevent or treat infection, or solutions that have similar composition to intracellular fluid are used. Irrigation may be used on open or closed wounds and requires sterile principles and technique in performing the procedure.

❧ ASSESSMENT

Type of wound and reason for irrigation, presence of infection, necrosis, or granulating tissue, type and amount of solution ordered and frequency of the treatment

❧ NURSING DIAGNOSES

High Risk for Infection; Impaired Tissue Integrity; Pain

❧ GOALS

Effective and safe wound irrigation provided; correct performance of the procedure and monitoring of wound healing

❧ INTERVENTIONS

Equipment/Supplies

- Sterile dressing set, gloves
- Sterile basins to hold solution and to receive irrigating solution from the wound
- Sterile dressings and tape if needed
- Petroleum jelly and tongue blade
- Sterile bulb or asepto syringe, 50 ml size
- Disposable gloves
- Sterile tubing or rubber tip for syringe
- Protective pads
- Sterile solution; normal saline, Ringer's solution, antibiotic solution

Resident

- Explain purpose of procedure and expected results
- Place in position of comfort, with area to be treated exposed and properly draped; protective cover or pad in place

❧ PROCEDURE

1. Perform handwashing.
2. Become familiar with the type of irrigation, solution, frequency of treatment ordered, type of dressings present.
3. Take the supplies to the bedside and identify the resident by wristband.
4. Warm solution to body temperature by placing in a pan of hot water and then pour in a sterile basin.
5. Remove the dressings using the clean disposable glove and place in proper disposal container; note skin and wound condition.
6. Draw up the solution from the basin into the syringe with dominant hand.

7. Direct the solution into the wound so all parts are filled from the cleanest to the least clean part and allow the solution to run into the basin held in place with nondominant hand under the wound.

8. Continue to draw up the solution and irrigate until about 200 ml is used.

9. Attach rubber tip or tube if inside of the wound is to be irrigated to prevent damage to the surrounding tissue.

10. Gently dry the skin around the wound with sterile gauze and apply petroleum jelly as a protective barrier.

11. Prepare the sterile dressing field; wash hands and put on sterile gloves to dress the wound if this is needed (see Wound Care, Dressing Change).

12. Discard used supplies according to universal precautions, store reusable supplies for next treatment if appropriate.

❧ PROBLEM-SOLVING ACTIONS

1. Avoid allowing any drainage from being drawn up into the syringe during the irrigation, holding syringe in a downward position will prevent this.

2. Irrigation may be continued until all drainage and debris have been removed.

3. Containers of solution should be capped, with name of resident and date opened written on the label.

4. Positioning varies with the site of the wound and need to place basin to receive the irrigating solution from the wound.

5. Other skin protector ointments may be used around the wound and applied with an applicator or gauze dressing.

6. If redressing is to be done, the sterile field may be set up initially and all the irrigating supplies placed on it with the dressings.

7. Wounds can be packed with Ringer's solution and dressed with hydrocolloid, thin-film polyurethane foam/membrane, or hydrogel dressings depending on the wound.

❧ EVALUATION

Successful performance of treatments without incident, progressive wound healing noted with absence of infectious process

WOUND CARE, SUTURE/STAPLE REMOVAL

Sutures or staples are surgical skin wound closures that are used to close or hold a wound together until healing is completed, usually 7 to 10 days following the procedure. Removal is timed during the healing process to prevent weakening or separation of a wound and unnecessary scar formation. It is timed based on the location and size of the incision, the age of the resident, and the presence of infection or drainage at the site. Skin sutures that are removable can be made of silk, synthetics, or wire (used for retention sutures to provide additional strength to the incision). Skin staples or clips are made of stainless steel and applied along the incisional line as an alternative to sutures to provide closure with minimal tissue response and scarring. All or selected sutures or staples can be removed at one time and adhesive skin Steri-Strips or butterfly-shaped adhesive closures applied to maintain wound closure and support the wound following the removal. General incisional cleansing precedes the removal and dressing change follows the removal using sterile technique (see Wound Care, Dressing Change).

ASSESSMENT

Number of days since surgery, age and medical status of the resident, presence of pain, redness, drainage or pus, wound edge approximation, type of sutures or staples

NURSING DIAGNOSES

High Risk for Infection; Body Image Disturbance; Impaired Skin Integrity

GOALS

Safe and correct removal of sutures or staples/clips provided without complications; wound closure maintained

INTERVENTIONS

Equipment/Supplies

- Sterile dressing set and suture or staple removal set
- Sterile dressings, gloves, tape individually wrapped as needed
- pH neutral cleansing agent
- Water proofed disposal bag

- Sterile scissors or staple remover
- Steri-Strips or butterfly adhesive closures
- Bath blanket for draping

Resident

- Explain purpose of procedure and expected results
- Place in position of comfort with draping of exposed incisional area

PROCEDURE

1. Perform handwashing.
2. Become familiar with type of wound closure and physician's order to remove all or some sutures or staples.

3. Provide proper light when assessing.

4. Set up sterile field; put sterile articles on field, open sterile gloves (see Wound Care, Dressing Change).

5. Situate the bag for disposal of used articles and dressings in a strategic position away from the field.

6. Remove the existing dressing and tape.

7. Put on sterile gloves and cleanse the suture line with antiseptic of any drainage or debris if the wound is clean and healing; a wound that is infected or gaping should be reported and no closures removed.

8. For suture removal:
    a. Grasp the knot with the forceps held in the nondominant hand and gently raise it away from the skin, cut the suture at the skin with the scissors held in the dominant hand and pull it up and out of the skin when removing the continuous sutures, discard the removed suture on the field or a gauze square.
    b. Cut each suture and remove to avoid contamination of the subcutaneous tissue depending on the type of the interrupted sutures.
    c. Remove every other or all of the interrupted sutures.
    d. To remove blanket continuous sutures, cut the suture on the side opposite of the loop stitch and draw the suture out in a steady direction of the loop with the forceps.
    e. Cut the suture and remove to avoid contamination of the subcutaneous tissue depending on the type of continuous sutures (mattress).
    f. Cleanse the incision with an antiseptic following removal of sutures.

9. For staple removal:
    a. Hold staple remover in the dominant hand and gently place the prongs under the staple.
    b. Gently close the instrument handles to allow for the third prong to close over the staple and press down to unbend the staple.
    c. Lift the instrument straight up and pull the staple from the skin.
    d. Discard staples as they are removed on the field or gauze square.
    e. Cleanse the incision with antiseptic following the removal of staples.

10. Apply Steri-Strips across the incision from the center outward to the upper and lower ends, then anchor these with two long strips applied to the full length on each side of the strips.

11. If butterfly closures are used, apply on the wound to provide support.

12. Dispose of all used articles and supplies according to Universal Precautions.

❧ PROBLEM SOLVING ACTIONS

1. Ensure that the resident does not have allergies to the antiseptic or tape removal solution.

2. Protect remaining sutures, staples, or butterfly or strip adhesive when bathing by covering the site with a waterproof material and taping in place like a picture frame.

3. Depending on the site of the incision, all or some of the sutures or staples can be removed.

4. If removal of the suture is difficult as in imbedded sutures or staples that have been left in place too long, notify the physician.

5. If Steri-Strips or butterfly adhesive tape is in place, refrain from cleansing over them when performing wound care as this could loosen and the support will be lost; apply tincture of benzoin to hold them in place.

❧ EVALUATION

Absence of inflammation or infectious process at the incisional site, wound clean, dry, intact, and healing following suture or staple removal

UNIT XIV

SPECIMEN PROCEDURES

- Blood Collection/Testing
- Feces Collection/Testing
- Urine Collection/Testing

BLOOD COLLECTION/TESTING

Blood collection and testing are done to determine the presence and abnormal amounts of constituents in the blood. Specimens are most commonly collected by capillary puncture or venipuncture. Venipuncture samples are collected from a vein in the antecubital space using a special collection device and vacuumized tubes known as Vacutainer. Capillary puncture samples are collected from the fingertip or ear lobe using a lancet to test for glucose with reagent strips or a glucose testing instrument (Glucoscan, Diascan, Accucheck, One Touch). This method of glucose testing, in most situations, has replaced urine testing for glucose as a means to determine the effective regulation of diabetes mellitus.

Agency testing for blood glucose, hemoglobin or microhematocult requires Clinical Laboratory Improvement Amendment (CLIA) certification or waiver certification.

❧ ASSESSMENT

Type of specimen collection and tests to be done, site to be used, frequency of glucose testing

❧ NURSING DIAGNOSES

High Risk for Infection; High Risk for Impaired Skin Integrity

❧ GOAL

Correct collection and accurate testing of blood specimen

❧ INTERVENTIONS

Equipment/Supplies

- Syringe/needle device, tubes with stoppers
- Glucoscan or other instrument
- Lancet in a device to perform finger stick
- Tourniquet
- Reagent test strips

- Antiseptic swabs
- Bandaid
- Gloves
- Plastic biohazard bag to transport specimen to the lab

Resident

- Explain purpose of procedure and expected results
- Place in sitting position with arm or hand supported

❧ PROCEDURE

1. Perform handwashing.
2. Assemble the equipment needed and become familiar with the site to be used and type of puncture and testing to be done.
3. Collect blood specimens by venipuncture:
   a. Apply the tourniquet to the upper arm above the site, put on gloves.
   b. Palpate the vein and cleanse with an alcohol swab allow to dry.
   c. Hold skin taut with nondominant hand and insert collecting device needle with the bevel side up at

a 15-45 degree angle.
   d. Insert the vacuum tube into the device with the dominant hand and push the tube inward to pierce the diaphragm.
   e. Note blood return in the tube and allow the tube to fill.
   f. Remove the tube and, with needle stabilized in the vein, continue to fill additional tubes as needed.
   g. Remove tourniquet after the tubes are filled and withdraw the needle as pressure is applied to the site with a small gauze square.
   h. Continue to apply pressure until bleeding has stopped, apply bandaid.
   i. Check and label the tubes and transport to the laboratory for ordered tests.
   j. Discard used articles according to Universal Precautions.

4. Collect and test blood specimens by capillary puncture:
   a. Request the resident to wash hands; put on gloves.
   b. Cleanse the fingertip or other site with alcohol swab and allow to dry.
   c. Puncture the side of a finger with the lancet holder and note bleeding.
   d. Squeeze the finger to obtain a drop of blood.
   e. With the instrument (Glucoscan) turned on, apply the blood to the reagent strip pad.
   f. When instrument indicates that it is ready, blot and press the strip pad down on the blotting paper and release after 2 seconds.
   g. Blot again on a clean area and note the colors on the paper made by each blot, apply pressure to the site.
   h. Open the door and insert the strip, close the door and, when the display indicates, note the glucose level displayed on the instrument.
   i. If using the One Touch, set the instrument to match the number on the test strip, slide the strip into the test strip holder in the instrument, secure the drop of blood by capillary puncture using the lancet device, apply the blood sample to the top of the test strip that is in the instrument, apply pressure to the site, wait for 45 seconds and read the printout on the instrument for the glucose level.
   j. Record the results on a flow sheet, discard used articles according to Universal Precautions.

❧ PROBLEM-SOLVING ACTIONS

1. Instructions are included in the many glucose monitoring instruments that are available and should be followed to ensure accurate results.

2. Perform timed glucose testing if needed and orders based on the results.

3. Use fresh reagent strips for tests.

4. Avoid using a cold or edematous finger to obtain capillary blood.

5. Avoid using arm with an intravenous or infectious skin site to obtain venous blood.

6. Note if coagulant therapy is received and maintain pressure at the site for at least 5 minutes following venipuncture.

7. Calibrate the unit used daily or according to the manufacturer's direction and record findings.

8. Gloves should be worn during all blood testing.

❧ EVALUATION

Collection and testing of blood for specific substances at the correct frequency; collection and transport of blood specimens to the laboratory for ordered tests

FECES COLLECTION/TESTING

Feces collection and testing screen for and detect abnormal constituents of the solid waste material eliminated from the large bowel. A specimen can be collected and sent to a laboratory for lipid and blood content and microorganism identification to obtain diagnostic information as well as the effectiveness of therapeutic interventions. Routine testing for occult blood can be done when gastrointestinal bleeding is suspected or needs to be monitored using a commercially prepared Hemoccult (Guaiac treated filter paper) test kit.

Agency testing for fecal occult blood requires Clinical Labortaory Improvement Amendment (CLIA) certification or waiver certification.

ASSESSMENT

Fecal characteristics (color, odor, consistency, mucus) dietary inclusion of meat or poultry, medications such as iron, Vitamin C, steroids, salicylate, iodides, rauwolfia, colchicine, and others that can affect test results

NURSING DIAGNOSES

Diarrhea; Constipation; Self-Care Deficit, Toileting

GOAL

Correct random or three time collection and testing of fecal material

INTERVENTIONS

Equipment/Supplies

- Hemoccult kit with slide packages and reagent solution
- Specimen container with a lid and label
- Bedpan and tongue depressor

- Disposable gloves
- Plastic biohazard bag if specimen transportation is necessary

Resident

- Explain purpose of procedure and expected results

PROCEDURE

1. Perform handwashing.
2. Inform the resident to use bedpan, commode, or toilet with a bedpan in place to defecate and not to discard toilet tissue in the pan with the feces.
3. Following defecation, remove the bedpan and put on gloves.
4. Provide or assist with anal cleaning.
5. With a tongue blade, remove a portion of the fecal material that includes any blood, mucus, or pus and place in a clean, plastic container and cover tightly with lid.
6. Label the container correctly and send to the laboratory while warm or place in the refrigerator to be transported at a later date.

7. Collect the number of specimens needed for confirmation of the findings.
8. Perform Hemoccult test:
    a. Collect the stool specimen as outlined above.
    b. Put on gloves.
    c. Open the flap on the side of the slide package.
    d. With an applicator, apply a small amount of the feces as a thin smear.
    e. Another thin smear of feces from another part of the specimen can also be done as some parts of the feces may not contain blood.
    f. Open flap in back of the slide with the smear and apply 2 drops of the solution on the paper containing the smears.
    g. Note the color change to blue indicating the presence of occult blood in the feces and record these results.

PROBLEM-SOLVING ACTIONS

1. Instructions are included with the commercial kit used for testing for occult blood that can be followed to ensure accurate results.
2. Consider and plan for timed specimen collection if ordered.
3. Hematest is another commercially prepared test to detect occult blood in feces.
4. Gloves should be worn during all feces testing.

EVALUATION

Collection and testing of feces for occult blood with results recorded; collection and transport of feces specimens to the laboratory for ordered tests

URINE COLLECTION/TESTING

Urine collection and testing are ordered to detect the presence and/or quantities of abnormal constituents in the urine. A specimen can be clean-catch for culture and microorganism identification, or can be random or aspirated from an indwelling catheter. It can be sent to a laboratory for routine analysis or other tests can be performed to obtain diagnostic information. Enzyme reagent strips or reagent tablets can be used to immediately obtain an estimate of the amount of a substance in the urine. The tests using reagent strips include glucose, ketones, protein, pH for acidity or alkalinity, and nitrite for bacteriuria with N-Multistix and include glucose, protein, ketones, and nitrite using Chemstrip. Diastix, Clinistix, and Tes-Tape are also reagent strips that are available to test for glucose in the urine. Clinitest and Acetest are reagent tablets to test for glucose and ketones respectively. Urine specific gravity can be determined by using an instrument called a urinometer, a calibrated hydrometer that measures the concentration of solutes in the urine if fluid and electrolyte imbalances are suspected.

Agency testing for urine glucose, ketones, nitrite, pH, specific gravity, or protein requires Clinical Laboratory Improvement Amendment (CLIA) certification or waiver certification.

✒ ASSESSMENT

Urinary elimination pattern, urine characteristics, signs and symptoms of urinary tract infection, I & O, presence of indwelling catheter, renal status and history of renal condition

✒ NURSING DIAGNOSES

High Risk for Infection; Altered Patterns of Urinary Elimination; High Risk for Fluid Volume Deficit

✒ GOAL

Correct collection and accurate testing of urine specimen

✒ INTERVENTIONS

Equipment/Supplies

- Bedpan or urinal
- Reagent tablet kit with test tube, dropper, tablets, and color chart

- Clean container and lid
- Graduated specimen container and urinometer

- Reagent strip, container, and color chart
- Toilet tissue

Resident

- Explain purpose of procedure and expected results

✒ PROCEDURE

1. Perform handwashing.
2. Inform the resident to use the bedpan, urinal, commode, or toilet with a bedpan in place to void and not to discard the toilet tissue in the pan with urine.

3. Following urination, put on gloves, remove the bedpan or urinal and pour 30-50 ml in a properly labeled clean plastic container and cover tightly with the lid to collect a random specimen to be sent to a lab; place in a clean container if urine is to be tested immediately with reagent strips or tablets.

4. Collect a double-voided specimen to test for glucose and ketones by requesting the resident to void, offer a glass of water and request to void again in 30 minutes, place both specimens in a clean container and test with reagent strips or tablets in the event that the resident is unable to void a second time.

5. Collect a specimen from an indwelling catheter by positioning the drainage tube to empty and clamp the tube distal to the specimen collection port; 15 minutes later, cleanse the port with an antiseptic swab and aspirate a urine sample with a 10 ml syringe and 21-25 gauge needle; place in a clean or sterile container for immediate or laboratory testing respectively.

6. Collect a clean-catch specimen by providing a kit and instructing to maintain the sterile inside of the container and to cleanse the meatus of the penis in a circular motion or labia and meatus in a front to back motion with soap and water or antiseptic solution provided; inform to start voiding, stop and continue to void in the container while holding the labia apart, carefully cover the labeled container without contamination of the inside lid or container.

7. Test urine with reagent strip or tape:
   a. Remove a strip from the container without touching the test end of the strip.
   b. Dip the test end in the random or second voided specimen for 2 seconds.
   c. Remove and tap away any excess urine against the side of the container.
   d. Time for 10-30 seconds depending on the strip used and hold the strip in air at eye level and compare the colors to the color chart on the container.
   e. Withdraw about 2 inches of tape from the dispenser roll and dip the end in the urine for 2 seconds, tap any excess urine against the container and hold at eye level for 60 seconds, compare to the color chart and wait and compare again in another 60 seconds if the first reading was positive.
   f. Record the results, discard the urine and rinse the container for reuse.

8. Test urine with reagent tablets:
   a. For Acetest, place a tablet on a piece of paper toweling and add 1 drop of a second voided urine specimen to the tablet.
   b. Wait 30 seconds and compare the color change, if any, to the color chart on the container or insert that comes with the kit.
   c. For Clinitest, place 5 drops of a second voided urine specimen in the test tube, rinse the dropper and add 10 drops of tap water.
   d. Place a tablet in the test tube, avoid touching the tablet if possible.
   e. Wait 15 seconds after the action in the solution stops and gently shake the tube avoid touching the sides of the tube.
   f. Compare the color of the solution with the color chart on the container or insert that comes with the kit.
   g. Record the results, discard the sample and wash, rinse, and air dry the articles for reuse, firmly replace lid on container of tablets.

9. Test urine with urinometer:
   a. Pour the urine into the cylinder until ¾ full.
   b. Gently place the calibrated urinometer into the cylinder of urine.
   c. Check to be sure that the instrument floats freely in the cylinder after the bobbling ceases.
   d. Read the specific gravity on the scale at the lowest part of the meniscus.
   e. Record the reading, discard the urine and cleanse and rinse the urinometer and the cylinder.

❧ PROBLEM-SOLVING ACTIONS

1. Instructions are included with the commercial kits used for testing urine that can be followed to ensure accurate results.

2. Timed specimens can also be collected for laboratory testing, usually 24 hours with or without a preservative, and requires information and instruction of the resident to cooperate with this lengthy collection.

3. Store reagent strips and tablets in a cool, dry place with the lid tightly closed, avoid using any discolored or outdated strips or tablets.

4. Test the urine specimen as soon after voiding as possible.

5. It is best to allow the urine to match room temperature before testing for specific gravity as this compares with the urinometer calibration.

6. Note medication regimen that can interfere with urine testing with reagent strips and affect results, such as levodopa, salicylates, and others, and use reagent tablets instead.

7. Gloves should be worn during all urine testing.

❧ EVALUATION

Collection and testing of urine for specific substances at the correct frequency on the proper type of specimen; transport of the specimen to a laboratory for ordered tests

UNIT XV

EMERGENCY PROCEDURES

- Cardiopulmonary Resuscitation
- Choking/Aspiration
- Resuscitation Bag

CARDIOPULMONARY RESUSCITATION

Cardiopulmonary resuscitation (CPR) is a method of providing systemic circulation by manual chest compression and oxygen by mouth-to-mouth breathing. The procedure is performed to prevent death following cardiac or pulmonary arrest, and once initiated, it is continued until spontaneous circulation and respirations are restored, or until emergency services assume responsibility for resuscitation. Unless resuscitation is initiated within 4-6 minutes, brain damage and/or death will occur. Cardiopulmonary resuscitation can be delivered by one or two persons. It is generally reserved for those who arrest unexpectedly or those with conditions that can cause an arrest. In residents with a terminal or irreversible disorder and in whom death is anticipated, an order can be written and recorded indicating that resuscitation should not be performed. This decision is identified by a "No Code" order that is documented on the chart. The decision for "No Code" is usually made by the physician and family members and can also be included in the resident's "advance directive."

Cardiopulmonary resuscitation is necessary when cardiac or pulmonary arrest occurs. Cardiac arrest is the cessation of the contractions necessary for circulation of blood to all parts of the body. It can be caused by heart failure, pulmonary embolus, myocardial infarction, or electrolyte imbalance (especially potassium). Pulmonary arrest is the cessation of air moving in and out of the lungs and the gas exchange process necessary to provide oxygen to the tissues and remove carbon dioxide. It can be caused by respiratory distress, airway obstruction, respiratory depression from trauma or drugs, or disorders affecting respiratory muscles. Complications that result from the procedure include rib fracture, mural thrombi or emboli, and abdominal distention.

❧ ASSESSMENT

Level of consciousness and ability to respond to stimuli, presence or absence of breathing, skin color, pupil response, presence or absence of a carotid pulse performed within 15 seconds

❧ NURSING DIAGNOSES

Decreased Cardiac Output; Altered Tissue Perfusion; Ineffective Breathing Pattern

❧ GOALS

To prevent a sudden death episode by establishing circulatory and respiratory function; correct delivery of cardiopulmonary resuscitation procedures

❧ INTERVENTIONS

Equipment/Supplies

- Arrest board

- Oropharyngeal airway

- Disposable pocket resuscitation mask with anti-reflux valve and oxygen adaptor

- Pre-inflated pocket resuscitation mask with anti-reflux valve and oxygen adaptor

<u>Resident</u>

- Position resident on a firm surface with head in proper alignment

❧ PROCEDURE

1. Shake shoulder and ask resident if he or she is alright.
2. Call for help and notify emergency services.
3. Place arrest board under the chest if resident is in bed or on the floor.
4. Note if airway obstructed and quickly remove any debris with a finger.
5. Position the head to open the airway:

   Head tilt method: Position a hand on the forehead and apply a firm, backward pressure to move the jaw forward to prevent the tongue from falling back into the pharynx.

   Head tilt with jaw thrust method: Place fingers of both hands at the angles of the jaw and move the lower jaw (mandible) forward and upward.

   Head tilt with chin lift method: Place hand on the forehead and tilt the head backward, place the fingers of the other hand on the mandible under the chin and move the chin forward.

6. Note the presence of respirations when the airway is opened by observing chest movement, place face or ear near the mouth and listen for or feel air on face.
7. If respirations are not present, maintain open airway with tilt chin or tilt neck lift method, pinch the nares closed, position protective equipment in place on the face, take a deep breath and place your mouth over the victim's mouth or place the disposable pocket resuscitation mask over the face with the breathing tube in place and perform 2 slow breaths (1 ½-2 seconds/breath) and observe the rise of the chest; allow for exhalation between breaths, quick ventilations; if a stoma is present, place mouth over the stoma to provide ventilations without positioning the head and neck.
8. Assess for absence of breathing and presence of carotid pulse, and if a pulse is present, deliver 1 breath every 5 seconds or 12/minute.
9. If pulse is not present, begin cardiac compression at a rate of 80-100/minute and in sequences of 15 compressions followed by 2 breaths, using the correct technique:
   a. Place fingers on lower rib margin and run fingers along the rib cage to the xiphoid process.
   b. Place the heel of the other hand on the sternum next to the fingers on the xiphoid process.
   c. Remove the fingers and place hand on top of the hand on the sternum and interlock the fingers in a position away from the rescuer.
   d. Maintain hand position and arms straight and do not move the hands from this position during the procedure.
10. Perform compressions of 1½ to 2 inches in depth to ensure blood flow while performing ventilations without interruption.
11. Assess the pulse and breathing following 1 minute (4 cycles of 15:2) of CPR, during a 5 second interruption, continue if there is no pulse present.
12. Continue to assess the pulse and breathing every few minutes for possible return of function.
13. If a second person is available for the procedure:
    a. Have rescuer kneel at side of victim on other side.
    b. First rescuer assesses pulse and, if absent, delivers 2 slow breaths and observes the rise of the chest.
    c. If no pulse, 5 compressions are delivered by the second rescuer to total 60/minute; followed by 1 slow breath by first rescuer.
    d. Continue with 2 rescuer method for 1 minute and check pulse; if no pulse present, continue with 5:1 cycle
    e. To switch positions, the first rescuer delivers one ventilation and moves to the position and prepares hands for compression; the pulse is assessed and ventilations resumed by the second rescuer at the same rate of 5:1 ratio of compressions to ventilations.

14. Continue procedure until assistance arrives or breathing and circulation is restored.

ᨒ PROBLEM-SOLVING ACTIONS

1. Have breathing bag and oxygen available, and connect O_2 to resuscitation bag or pocket mask and set at 10-15 L/min.; administer oxygen when ventilation and circulation have been restored.

2. Provide emergency services with all important information about resident's condition.

3. Compressor calls for switch. Compressor completes 5th compression. Ventilator completes ventilation, then switches.

4. A disposable pocket resuscitation mask should be positioned on the face to give complete protection to the rescuer as it keeps the hands, face, and mouth from coming in contact with the victim's breath and body fluids; it is a one piece plastic unit that covers the whole face and has a one-way valve in the breathing tube to allow for the inflow of air. If a mask is not readily available, do not delay the administration of CPR.

5. An alternative pocket resuscitation mask that maintains the airway is a pre-inflated, contoured, and made of plastic to fit over the face; it allows no backflow of air or fluids. It is prepared and used as follows:
   a. Remove from the carrying case.
   b. Push out the dome of the mask.
   c. Mount the one-way valve on the mask port.
   d. Position head backwards and place the mask on the face over the open mouth and nose.
   e. Clamp mask to face and hold in place with hands on each side.
   f. Blow through mouthpiece until the chest rises.

ᨒ EVALUATION

Breathing and pulse re-established

CHOKING/ASPIRATION

Choking and aspiration are common problems in the older adult. Choking is usually the result of chewing and swallowing (dysphagia) dysfunctions and can lead to aspiration. Chewing can be affected by poorly-fitted dentures. Dysphagia can be related to unconscious states, disorders that cause a loss of or diminished swallowing reflex, or a decrease in muscle strength. Chewing and swallowing dysfunctions increase the possibility of aspiration of foods, fluids, saliva, mucus and other secretions. Inability to chew and swallow effectively allows for accumulation of foods and fluid and aspiration into the trachea since the separation between the airway and the esophagus is rendered inadequate when swallowing is inadequate.

Aspiration can also be caused by cardiopulmonary resuscitation (CPR) or enteral feedings. Either can result in regurgitation of stomach contents or formula by reflux into the esophagus leading to aspiration and entry into the trachea. CPR that causes gastric distention reduces the pressure over the gastroesophageal spinchter allowing for reflux, and if the head of the bed is not raised during and after tube feedings, reflux of the formula into the esophagus and aspiration can result.

Complications of aspiration and associated difficulties include aspiration pneumonia and malnutrition.

❧ ASSESSMENT

Ability to cough, chew, and swallow, a fluctuating level of consciousness, drooling, accumulations of secretions in the oral cavity, inability to talk or breathe during choking

❧ NURSING DIAGNOSES

Ineffective Airway Clearance, High Risk for Aspiration; Altered Nutrition: Less Than Body Requirements; Impaired Swallowing

❧ GOALS

Control of coughing, choking, chewing, and swallowing activities; correct preventive interventions to reduce possible aspiration

❧ INTERVENTIONS

Equipment/Supplies

- Suctioning equipment and supplies
- Disposable gloves
- Resuscitation bag and oxygen if needed

Resident

- Explain purpose of assessments and procedure and expected results
- Place in semi-Fowler's position for feedings and with head turned to the side depending on level of consciousness

❧ PROCEDURE

1. Perform handwashing.

2. Become familiar with the ability to swallow and the possibility of coughing or choking while eating or drinking.

3. Facilitate eating by offering soft-textured foods and note ability to chew and swallow and motor control of the lips and tongue.

4. Maintain the head in an elevated position without hyperextension of the neck.

5. Note any accumulation of food or secretions and suction as needed (see Suctioning).

6. Allow time for chewing and swallowing small amounts of food or fluid during meals.

7. To remove airway obstruction in a conscious/unconscious resident:
   a. Assess for universal choking and signal of individual grasping at their throat.
   b. Administer 5 manual thrusts.
   c. Repeat thrusts until effective or resident becomes unconscious.
   d. If unconscious, activate emergency system. Perform tongue-jaw lift and finger sweep the oral cavity to remove any foreign material, try to ventilate and give up to 5 manual thrusts, repeat procedure until effective.

PROBLEM-SOLVING ACTIONS

1. If resident is choking, allow to cough up the substance(s) before attempting to remove by other methods.

2. Poor fitting dentures should be corrected to facilitate chewing.

3. Perform tracheal suctioning if oropharyngeal suctioning is ineffective in removing and clearing substances from the throat and airway.

EVALUATION

Absence of aspiration or airway obstruction associated with chewing and swallowing dysfunction

RESUSCITATION BAG

Resuscitation bag (Ambu) is utilized for manual restoration of ventilation in individuals experiencing respiratory arrest. It is used to provide room air or oxygen as well as promote ventilation during or after cessation of breathing and, if available, can be utilized during cardiopulmonary resuscitation.

ASSESSMENT

Respiratory status that includes length of time since breathing ceased, resident condition or circumstances requiring manual ventilatory support

NURSING DIAGNOSES

Ineffective Breathing Pattern, Altered Tissue Perfusion; Ineffective Airway Clearance

GOALS

Ventilation established with tissue oxygenation; correct use of hand-held breathing bag

INTERVENTIONS

Equipment/Supplies

- Resuscitation bag
- Oropharyngeal airway
- Oxygen and tubing connected to wall or tank
- Oxygen adapter and flowmeter
- Suction equipment and supplies

Resident

- Place in supine position with head in proper alignment

PROCEDURE

1. Perform handwash if time allows.
2. Assess airway for objects or debris and remove with finger.
3. Determine if this causes breathing to return and, if not, insert an oropharyngeal airway if available.
4. Place one hand on the back of the neck and move jaw forward with the other hand to prevent tongue from falling back and obstructing pharynx.
5. Connect the bag to O_2 at 10-15 L/minute and place the mask that is attached to the breathing bag over the nose and mouth.
6. Place pressure on the mask to seal to the face and prevent any air from escaping.
7. Compress the bag with one hand while holding the mask in place with the other hand.
8. Perform one compression of the bag every 5 seconds.
9. Note that the chest should rise and fall with each compression.
10. If manual resuscitation via a breathing bag is performed on a tracheostomy, place the bag directly over the stoma or attach it directly to the tube that is present.
11. Continue compression until ventilation is restored and returns to normal.

❧ PROBLEM-SOLVING ACTIONS

1. Reassess placement of mask on face if chest fails to rise and fall during manual resuscitation with the breathing bag.

2. If oxygen is administered, connect the tubing from the oxygen source to the breathing bag and turn the oxygen on to the appropriate setting (10-15 L/minute).

3. Vomitus or accumulated mucus can be removed by oropharyngeal suctioning before or during the procedure to maintain an open airway.

❧ EVALUATION

Respirations established and returned to baseline range

UNIT XVI

PSYCHOSOCIAL PROCEDURES

- Behavior Management
- Cognitive Enhancement
- Communication Facilitation
- Environmental Safety
- Relaxation Therapy
- Socialization Facilitation
- Spiritual Facilitation
- Therapeutic Activities

BEHAVIOR MANAGEMENT

Behavior management includes the management of anger, confusion, hallucinations and other behavior by utilizing techniques such as area limitations, self-responsibility, group interactions, limit setting, and behavior modifications depending on individual needs. Behavior changes can be attributed to dementia disorders or psychological conflicts resulting from a loss of control over body, environment, and unmet needs such as pain, hunger, thirst, and toileting. They may include combativeness, arguing, agitation, and aggressiveness.

❧ ASSESSMENT

Behavior manifestation and cause, history of mental, emotional or physiologic disorders that contribute to behavior, medications taken to control behavior

❧ NURSING DIAGNOSES

Anxiety; Ineffective Individual Coping; Hopelessness; Impaired Social Interaction; Altered Thought Processes; High Risk for Violence Directed at Others

❧ GOALS

Modification of behavior for optimal functioning and well-being

❧ INTERVENTIONS

None

❧ PROCEDURE

1. Establish rapport with calm approach and supportive attitude.
2. Monitor for inappropriate behavior and intervene before harmful, combative, or frustrated behavior is expressed.
3. Allow for expression of anger while establishing limits and informing individual of consequences of behavior.
4. Identify desired behaviors and assist to achieve these in appropriate situations.
5. Refrain from punitive actions or arguing with resident about behavior.
6. Use support group or therapeutic group to provide emotional support and information about behavioral changes.
7. Note behaviors that indicate hallucinations or delusions and assist to maintain reality-based thought process and to define and acknowledge reality as opposed to other thinking and behavior.
8. Avoid unfamiliar situations and decision making responsibility of individual.
9. Provide structure with routines and low to moderate stimulation in the environment.
10. Implement cognitive management if individual is confused or disoriented.
11. Utilize physical restraints by physician order or restrict to an area if indicated, allow wandering for those with dementia to prevent frustration or anger; utilize an alarm system in order to monitor location and prevent harmful situations.
12. Assist to replace undesirable behavior with desirable behavior and praise all efforts for behavior change.

13. Develop and facilitate a behavior modification program:
    a. Assist individual to record behaviors to be changed.
    b. Reinforce changes to acceptable behaviors and attempts at self-control.
    c. Withdraw praise and reinforcement when behaviors are undesirable.
    d. Offer reinforcers that work for the individual, such as, attention, points or merits, special treats, small gifts, applause.
    e. Provide reinforcers immediately following desired behavior and administer only when behavior is changed.

14. Provide diversion or redirect attention away from aggressive or agitated behaviors.

15. Provide an environment that allows the individual to be held responsible for their own behavior by giving them as much control as possible.

16. Provide "time out" periods if necessary.

❧ PROBLEM-SOLVING ACTIONS

1. Administer psychotropic drugs as ordered and evaluate for possible reduced dosage or discontinuation.

2. Provide appropriate supervision and assistance to those who are chronically confused or have irreversible neurologic deficits.

3. Utilize mental and physical aids to minimize frustration and enhance self-responsibility.

4. Provide a role model by own expressions and behavior.

5. Determining possible causes of the behavior such as excessive external stimulation in the environment, deprivation of basic needs and take steps to correct the problem to control the behavior.

6. Behavior management of catastrophic reaction, violence, extreme combativeness, paranoia, and halucinations require special psychiatric techniques and confinement.

❧ EVALUATION

Behavior change facilitated with expression of anger and negative behaviors and responses managed in a constructive fashion; compliance with behavior modification program with behavioral expectations achieved; resident calmer and less combative and confused

COGNITIVE ENHANCEMENT

Cognitive management includes a combination of mental stimulation, reality orientation, and memory training. It is done to enable an individual to comprehend and develop awareness of their environment and sense of self and others. It includes reminiscence therapy and validation therapy to promote memory and communication. Those who benefit from this treatment include individuals that experience a disruption in cognitive abilities and activities. Disorders such as Alzheimer's disease, organic brain syndrome, dementia, and neurologic conditions that affect thinking, memory, orientation, attention span, reasoning, decision-making, ability to follow directions, and problem-solving as well as change in affect and sleep patterns cause difficulty in adaption to circumstances within the environment. This leads to dysfunctional or undesirable thinking and behaviors.

❧ ASSESSMENT

Mental and emotional status, orientation to time, person, place, and events, degree of memory and judgment impairment, history of dementia-type disorder or other condition affecting cognitive functioning

❧ NURSING DIAGNOSES

Altered Thought Processes; Sleep Pattern Disturbance, Impaired Social Interaction

❧ GOALS

Improved cognitive status with increased personal awareness of environment and circumstances

❧ INTERVENTIONS

None

❧ PROCEDURE

1. Provide stimulation gradually or as tolerated throughout the waking hours (interaction with staff members and other residents, newspapers, calendars, radios, music, books, familiar personal objects, family members and friends).

2. Present information in both written and oral forms using repetition when needed.

3. Use reminders such as color coding on drawers, labeling items, checklists, notes.

4. Remind of thoughts expressed to stimulate memory.

5. Inform resident of altered thinking in an unthreatening way, such as, personalization, generalization, memory loss, irrational judgment.

6. Encourage expression of past events and feelings; encourage writing about them if desired.

7. Focus on past experiences if distracted or unable to maintain attention span.

8. Facilitate recall of past by repeating sessions, commenting on the importance of the past, using effective communication techniques.

9. Provide consistency in care, staff, and situations or inform of change prior to its implementation to prevent disorientation and frustration.

10. Maintain an approach that is calm, familiar and reflects the capability of the individual.

11. Utilize techniques to train memory, such as games, lists, tags, information repetition, association clues, pictures, group programs, others.

12. Encourage memory of recent events by discussing, asking questions.

13. Assist to repeat and rehearse noting the time, date, and activity at specific times of the day.

PROBLEM-SOLVING ACTIONS

1. Limit decision making and directions that will frustrate the resident.

2. Limit stimuli if disorientation is increased by over-stimulation or confusion is created.

3. Provide realistic situations in daily living routines to focus on and practice orientation facilitation.

4. Attempt new learning experiences to promote and train memory if appropriate.

5. Use touch, if appropriate, to stimulate awareness.

EVALUATION

Cognitive status facilitated and improved; awareness and thought process maintained at optimal level based on progression of the disorder

COMMUNICATION FACILITATION

Communication is facilitated by active listening, hearing, verbalizing, and visualizing verbal and non-verbal messages, any of which can be affected by the aging process or disease. The communication process enhances interpersonal interaction necessary for socialization and informing staff of needs and desires. It is also important for staff in order to interpret behavior and care for residents with speech or language disturbances, hearing or visual deficits. Art therapy is a method that facilitates communication through drawings to determine behavior, feelings, and thoughts about stressful events or environment, and relationships. The use of alternative communication methods should be planned and decided with the resident to promote adaptation to the device or behavior change.

❧ ASSESSMENT

Presence of visual or auditory deficits, dysarthria, aphasia, need for alternate methods for communication, medical or surgical interventions that create communication deficits

❧ NURSING DIAGNOSES

Sensory/Perceptual Alterations; Impaired Verbal Communications; Ineffective Individual Coping; High Risk for Trauma

❧ GOALS

Communication enhanced by use of alternate methods to correct impairments and develop communication skills; correct use and care of hearing and visual aids

❧ INTERVENTIONS

Equipment/Supplies

- Eye glasses, contact lenses, case for storage
- Hearing aid, batteries, if needed
- Cleansing materials for glasses, contacts

Resident

- Explain purpose of procedure and expected results

❧ PROCEDURE

1. Listen attentively to what resident says with interest, eliminate distractions from the environment.
2. Observe nonverbal behavior for messages indicating feelings and thoughts.
3. Clarify communications by using feedback to ensure understanding of messages.
4. Provide a comfortable noise-free environment and sitting or other position in proximity that enhances communication, hearing, and vision of resident and staff member.
5. For visual impairment:
   a. Communicate your presence by speaking to or touching the resident.
   b. Familiarize the resident with items in the room and describe furniture and articles in the room, avoid moving or changing placement or location of articles.
   c. Assist with meals, if needed, and walking in unfamiliar places.

  d. Provide magnifying glass, large print materials, Braille reading material.
  e. Provide access to glasses and contacts, clean when needed.

6. For auditory impairment:
  a. Use appropriate voice volume when speaking to the resident.
  b. Provide paper and pencil, slate or other methods to communicate.
  c. Provide access to hearing aids that fit in the ear or are placed in a pocket, clean and replace batteries when needed.
  d. Face the resident when speaking to promote lip reading.
  e. Provide sound enhancement for telephone.

7. For speech impairment:
  a. Provide communication aids such as paper and pencil, slate, picture board or cards, or other methods to assist resident in making needs known.
  b. Encourage to repeat words or sentences and practice sounds and speech patterns.
  c. Have patience and avoid rushing resident to speak or respond.
  d. Obtain an interpreter, if needed, for those who do not speak English or for those for whom English is a second language.

8. For art therapy:
  a. Provide art supplies needed to draw or paint and space to work.
  b. Offer encouragement and support to express feelings in the art work.
  c. Remain with resident while painting or drawing and observe behavior and listen to conversations or descriptions regarding the art work.
  d. Avoid interpreting the art work unless combined with long-term art for comparisons and assessment data.

9. Engage in communication with resident using short sentences and understandable words, and offer one request, reminder, or direction at a time to avoid causing misunderstandings and frustration.

10. Monitor own body language when communicating with resident.

❧ PROBLEM-SOLVING ACTIONS

1. Provide access to a speech pathologist, occupational therapist, audiologist, ophthalmologist, and transportation for evaluation, if needed.

2. Instruct resident in care of visual and hearing aids and safe storage of these devices if resident is receptive and able to perform activities.

❧ EVALUATION

Communication facilitated regardless of deficits; communication, visual, auditory, speech aids utilized effectively

ENVIRONMENTAL SAFETY

Environmental safety includes the management and prevention of risks of abuse (verbal, emotional, and physical), trauma and physical injury, mental and physical comfort (temperature, personal hygiene, rest, lighting, humidity, stimulation). Manipulation of the environment and behavior changes by the staff members are required to provide safety and security for the residents.

❧ ASSESSMENT

Presence of environmental hazards, complaints about the environment and/or staff members, cleanliness, presence of physical injury noted, combative behavior, history of insomnia or perceptual deficits

❧ NURSING DIAGNOSES

High Risk for Traumas; Impaired Physical Mobility, Sensory/Perceptual Alterations; Altered Thought Processes; Violence Potential: Self-Directed or Directed at Others

❧ GOALS

Identification of environmental hazard and modifications to maintain safety and security of residents

❧ INTERVENTIONS

None

❧ PROCEDURE

1. Remove environmental hazards such as throw rugs, cluttered pathways, spills on floor, wet floors, furniture that doesn't lock.
2. Position articles within reach to avoid need to reach.
3. Provide hand rails or side rails as needed.
4. Provide a roommate with similar needs and one who has rapport with resident.
5. Adjust room temperature, humidity to optimal level; avoid exposure to drafts or heat.
6. Adjust lighting to optimal level; avoid glare or direct light in eyes.
7. Control noise level if necessary.
8. Provide personal care and clean bed with proper blankets and pillows for positioning and comfort.
9. Utilize restraints and monitor according to agency policy and physician orders.
10. Provide surveillance of resident and staff interactions if abuse is suspected and monitor for signs of resident abuse.
11. Restrict visitors and limit stimulation in the environment if needed.
12. Provide consistency in daily care and staff according to resident request if possible.

❧ PROBLEM-SOLVING ACTIONS

1. If a resident is at risk for injury, remove him/her from the environment or modify to ensure safety.
2. Take proper steps to prevent or report staff abuses of residents.
3. Carry out fire drills and fire prevention measures according to agency policy.

4. Ensure proper equipment maintenance and pest control to ensure resident safety.

5. Place a sign on broken equipment and remove from resident's area; notify the maintenance department or appropriate individual.

❧ EVALUATION

Absence of physical, mental, or emotional injury; safe environment maintained in compliance with resident needs

RELAXATION THERAPY

Relaxation therapy includes a combination of techniques such as calming, guided imagery, music, meditation, biofeedback, distraction, and the use of support group therapy to reduce pain, anxiety and fear, and promote adaptation to the environment. Methods are selected based on individual needs, desires, and a history of what has worked in the past.

❧ ASSESSMENT

Mental and emotional status and level of anxiety, reason for anxiety, use of coping skills and defense mechanisms, possible need for counseling to reduce anxiety, medications taken to control anxiety

❧ NURSING DIAGNOSES

Anxiety, Fatigue, Chronic Pain, Fear, Ineffective Individual Coping, Powerlessness, Sleep Pattern Disturbance

❧ GOALS

Reduction in anxiety or uneasiness by effective use of relaxation techniques

❧ INTERVENTIONS

Equipment/Supplies

- Music cassettes, compact discs, radio, television
- Relaxation tapes for breathing or muscle techniques
- Tape player (portable with ear phones)

Resident

- Explain purpose of the activity and expected results
- Place in position of comfort in a quiet environment

❧ PROCEDURE

1. Establish rapport and trusting relationship with a calm, supportive attitude.
2. Control stimuli in the environment and create a noise free, stress free atmosphere when relaxation techniques are implemented.
3. Use touch, hand holding, and backrub to promote relaxation when appropriate.
4. Provide diversional activities and distraction, such as, humor, imagery, music, or centering to focus attention from the source of anxiety.
5. Encourage slow and deep breathing with eyes closed and lying or sitting in a relaxed position.
6. Remain with resident and allow for expressions of feelings and concerns.
7. Provide music cassettes or compact discs with ear phones in a quiet room; radio or TV music or relaxation programs can also be used.
8. Allow for quiet time and regulate visitations according to anxiety level and needs.
9. Provide for meditation and/or yoga:
   a. Provide a quite space with room to lie down or sit in a chair.
   b. Advise to close eyes and relax all muscles.

   c. Inform to select a word and to repeat it and focus on it during expiration; a word such as "you" or "me" may be used.

   d. Continue this for the desired length of time and when finished, open eyes and remain quiet for a few minutes.

   e. Advise to return to the procedure when needed.

   f. Provide a mat on the floor to perform yoga movements and positions, if desired.

10. Provide for guided imagery:

   a. Provide a quiet environment and advise to close eyes and sit or lie in a comfortable position.

   b. Suggest that the individual think of a pleasant experience from the past.

   c. Allow the individual to describe the experience and guide the images with a soft voice by making. suggestions about the images such as floating, sensory experiences of the imagery such as smell, taste, sight, hearing, and feeling.

   d. Assist in termination of the imagery by suggesting counting or deep breathing and advise on frequency of practicing imagery.

11. Provide for relaxation therapy:

   a. Provide a quiet environment conducive to relaxation, such as, reduced lighting, noise-free, comfortable temperature, comfortable clothing, comfortable area for sitting or lying positions.

   b. Use low voice and pace words according to activity.

   c. Describe techniques and allow to perform deep breathing, abdominal breathing, or imagery.

   d. Using a tape and earphones or vocal instruction, request to tense all muscles for a few minutes and then relax all muscles slowly; then, in sequence from toes, feet, legs, abdomen, buttocks, arms, fingers, hands, neck, and facial muscles, tense each muscle or muscle group and slowly relax each one while deep breathing.

   e. Inform that it is essential to concentrate on the technique used to achieve a sense of relaxation.

   f. Assist in termination of the muscle relaxation and suggest repeating the procedure independently.

12. Encourage participation in a support group that focuses on anxiety reduction.

❧ PROBLEM-SOLVING TECHNIQUES

1. Administer anti-anxiety drugs as ordered and evaluate for possibility of reduced dosages or discontinuation as relaxation therapy is instituted.

2. Provide a role model for relaxation by own behavior and attitude.

3. Determine need and arrange for biofeedback to treat pain or anxiety or manage stress as an alternative to other relaxation techniques.

❧ EVALUATION

Resident practices selected relaxation techniques; anxiety reduced to optimal level as support and relaxation are achieved

SOCIALIZATION FACILITATION

*S*ocialization is facilitated by group activities, recreational therapy and the encouragement
of visits by family and friends that are beneficial to the resident. The activities should be
selected to enhance social skills according to individual capabilities. The availability of a
recreational therapist allows for planned activities to reduce anxiety, stimulate sensory percep-
tions, as well as enhance socialization and relaxation. Some facilities include programs
arranged with community groups such as children's visits and correspondence exchanges, pet
visits, and entertainment groups.

ASSESSMENT

Family participation and interest in visitation and involvement in care planning, preferences in activities and level of participation, presence of physical, psychological, mental, or social deficits,
preferences and need for visitation; need for group activities or therapy

NURSING DIAGNOSES

Diversional Activity Deficit; Chronic Pain; Sensory/Perceptual Alterations; Impaired Social
Interaction; Social Isolation

GOALS

Purposeful socialization with improved social skills and acceptance of and participation in planned
group activities and recreation

INTERVENTIONS

None

PROCEDURE

1. Encourage to identify and participate in activities with another individual or in groups.

2. Provide a list of activities available within and outside the facility.

3. Inform of the importance of recreation and interactions without blaming or placing pressure and guilt
   on the individual.

4. Provide a positive view and reinforcement for participation and note responses, such as smiling,
   laughing, relaxation, stimulation, personal satisfaction, fatigue.

5. Maintain a safe environment and one that is relaxed and nonjudgmental when obtaining activities for
   individual or group participation.

6. Select activities appropriate for age and abilities.

7. Provide comfortable space and privacy for visits from family and friends.

8. Facilitate programs for children, music, theater groups to visit and perform.

9. Provide telephone and mailing services when desired.

10. Allow for flexible visiting schedules, limit visitation time when appropriate to ensure rest for the
    individual and provide a rationale for the visitor.

11. Include family in social groups and activities when possible.

❧ PROBLEM-SOLVING ACTIONS

1. Provide access to recreational therapist, activity director, rehabilitation nurse aide, physical therapist or occupational therapist for therapeutic program to reduce anxiety and improve social skills.

2. Provide a roommate with similar interests and age.

3. Provide access and transportation to entertainment activities outside the facility.

❧ EVALUATION

Increased participation in social activities and recreation; friendships and relationships established; positive response from planned program to enhance social skills

SPIRITUAL FACILITATION

The presence or absence of religious beliefs are important considerations in the care of residents. Each person's beliefs and practices should be respected and accepted. Every effort should be made to fulfill them. They may include religious rituals, dietary requirements, or health practices. For those who do not wish to participate in formal religious events or practices, the same recognition and respect for their wishes and rights should be fulfilled.

ASSESSMENT

Religious preference and expressed desire to participate in religious practices, need for counseling and visits from clergy

NURSING DIAGNOSES

Spiritual Distress

GOALS

Spiritual needs and care identified and implemented

INTERVENTIONS

None

PROCEDURE

1. Provide transportation to church or synagogue in the community or to the chapel in the facility on the Sabbath, special religious holidays, or when requested.

2. Provide space and allow for religious articles, such as Bible, rosary, other symbols.

3. Arrange for special dietary inclusion and restrictions per resident request.

4. Prepare for special ritual experiences in room, such as communion, anointing of the sick, or other procedures, and ensure privacy.

5. Arrange visit by the appropriate clergy if requested.

6. Allow the resident to express spiritual needs, and whether religion is accepted or rejected by resident.

7. Avoid imposing own beliefs on the resident.

PROBLEM-SOLVING ACTIONS

1. Observe resident for nonverbal behavior indicating the need or desire for spiritual counseling.

2. Allow for alternatives to traditional practices of medical care, such as, Christian Science practitioner, faith healing, naturalistic health, laying on of hands, others.

3. Follow appropriate religious care of resident who is terminal or in treatment after death according to resident or family request.

EVALUATION

Participation in religious activities as desired

THERAPEUTIC ACTIVITIES

Therapeutic activities assist the resident to appreciate, express, and perceive feelings and thoughts to achieve a sense of well-being. They may include animal therapy to provide affection, music therapy to provide relaxation, humor to provide diversion and relieve tension, and touch to provide caring and comfort. Activities preferred by the individual result in behavior change that allows for relaxation, enhanced coping ability, learning facilitation, and the ability to socialize and establish relationships with others. Individual considerations should be made for those who do not wish to participate in planned activities.

ASSESSMENT

Preference for activities and expressed desire to participate, need for therapeutic interventions and specific activities to offer

NURSING DIAGNOSES

Anxiety; Ineffective Individual Coping, Diversional Activity Deficit, Sensory/Perceptual Alterations, Impaired Social Interaction

GOALS

Therapeutic activities provided with positive behavior and attitude changes indicating improved psychosocial status

INTERVENTIONS

Equipment/Supplies

- Music cassettes, compact discs

- Radio, television

- Various animals from community agencies that have been inspected and approved by health officials

Resident

- Explain purpose of the activity and expected results

- Place in position of comfort in a quiet environment or in a small group

PROCEDURE

1. Provide visits of animals such as dogs, cats, birds.

2. Encourage resident to hold and pet the animals; play with and speak to the pets.

3. Arrange for pets to visit daily or as frequently as possible if resident wishes.

4. Provide music cassettes or compact discs with small portable recorder and ear phones and provide selections preferred by the resident and dependent on desired change in behavior.

5. Maintain a noise-free environment and proper volume of music.

6. Provide music via the radio or television for visual and auditory stimulation and monitor length of time music is playing.

7. Allow resident to play an instrument if able and desired.

8. Encourage smiles and laughter from resident and respond in a positive manner for approval.

9. Interact with resident by supplying type of humor that elicits response.

10. Provide fun games, cartoons, books, and jokes based on resident preference and what arouses laughter.

11. Encourage to tell jokes and silly stories or relate funny past experiences.

12. Inform of humorous situations within the environment.

13. Touch resident on arm or shoulder at times of stress, pain, or other discomforts; hold hand if fearful and during periods of extreme anxiety.

❧ PROBLEM-SOLVING ACTIONS

1. Check and maintain working order of music equipment.

2. Refrain from using touch if resident rejects this intervention.

3. Allow participation in therapeutic activities alone or in group as preferred.

4. Allow pet to remain with and receive care from the resident if possible, such as, bird in a cage, aquarium of fish.

❧ EVALUATION

Change in feelings and behavior observed, tension relieved, socialization and relaxation facilitated, positive response to humor

APPENDIX A

The 1992-93 List of NANDA Nursing Diagnoses*

- Activity Intolerance
- Activity Intolerance, High Risk for
- Adjustment, Impaired
- Airway Clearance, Ineffective
- Anxiety
- Aspiration, High Risk for
- Body Image Disturbance
- Body Temperature, High Risk for Altered
- Breastfeeding, Effective
- Breastfeeding, Ineffective
- Breastfeeding, Interrupted
- Breathing Pattern, Ineffective
- Cardiac Output, Decreased
- Caregiver Role Strain
- Caregiver Role Strain, High Risk for
- Communication, Impaired Verbal
- Constipation
- Constipation, Colonic
- Constipation, Perceived
- Coping, Defensive
- Coping, Ineffective Individual
- Decisional Conflict (Specify)
- Denial, Ineffective
- Diarrhea
- Disuse Syndrome, High Risk for
- Diversional Activity Deficit
- Dysfunctional Ventilatory Weaning Response
- Dysreflexia
- Family Coping, Compromised, Ineffective
- Family Coping, Disabling, Ineffective
- Family Coping, Potential for Growth
- Family Processes, Altered
- Fatigue

- Fear
- Fluid Volume Deficit
- Fluid Volume Deficit, High Risk for
- Fluid Volume Excess
- Gas Exchange, Impaired
- Grieving, Anticipatory
- Grieving, Dysfunctional
- Growth and Development, Altered
- Health Maintenance, Altered
- Health-Seeking Behaviors (Specify)
- Home Maintenance Management, Impaired
- Hopelessness
- Hyperthermia
- Hypothermia
- Incontinence, Bowel
- Incontinence, Functional
- Incontinence, Reflex
- Incontinence, Stress
- Incontinence, Total
- Incontinence, Urge
- Infant Feeding Pattern, Ineffective
- Infection, High Risk for
- Injury, High Risk for
- Knowledge Deficit (Specify)
- Management of Therapeutic Regime (Individual), Ineffective
- Noncompliance (Specify)
- Nutrition: Less than Body Requirements, Altered
- Nutrition: More than Body Requirements, Altered
- Nutrition: Potential for More than Body Requirements, Altered
- Oral Mucous Membrane, Altered
- Pain

- Pain, Chronic
- Parental Role Conflict
- Parenting, Altered
- Parenting, High Risk for Altered
- Peripheral Neurovascular Dysfunction, High Risk for
- Personal Identity Disturbance
- Physical Mobility, Impaired
- Poisoning, High Risk for
- Post-Trauma Response
- Powerlessness
- Protection, Altered
- Rape-Trauma Syndrome
- Rape-Trauma Syndrome: Compound Reaction
- Rape Trauma Syndrome: Silent Reaction
- Relocation Stress Syndrome
- Role Performance, Altered
- Self-Care Deficit: Bathing/Hygiene, Dressing/Grooming, Feeding, Toileting
- Self-Esteem, Chronic Low
- Self-Esteem, Situational Low
- Self-Esteem Disturbance
- Self Mutilation, High Risk for
- Sensory/Perceptual Alterations (Specify: Visual, Auditory, Kinesthetic, Gustatory, Tactile, Olfactory)
- Sexual Dysfunction
- Sexual Patterns, Altered
- Skin Integrity, Impaired
- Skin Integrity, High Risk for
- Sleep Pattern Disturbance
- Social Interaction, Impaired
- Social Isolation
- Spiritual Distress (Distress of the Human Spirit)
- Suffocation, High Risk for
- Swallowing, Impaired
- Thermoregulation, Ineffective
- Thought Processes, Altered

- Tissue Integrity, Impaired
- Tissue Perfusion, Altered (Specify Type: Renal, Cerebral, Cardiopulmonary, Gastrointestinal, Peripheral)
- Trauma, High Risk for
- Unilateral Neglect
- Urinary Elimination, Altered
- Urinary Retention
- Ventilation, Inability to Sustain Spontaneous
- Violence, High Risk for: Self-Directed or Directed at Others

NANDA is the North American Nursing Diagnosis Association

APPENDIX B

REFERENCES

Centers for Disease Control. (1986). Recommendations for preventing transmission of infection. *Morbidity and Mortality Weekly Report, 35*.

La Rocca, J.C. and Otto, S.E. (1992). *Pocket guide to intravenous therapy* (2nd ed.). St. Louis: Mosby-Year Book.

Lewis, S.M. and Collier, I.C. (1992). *Medical-surgical nursing: assessment and management of clinical problems* (3rd ed.). St. Louis: Mosby-Year Book.

Lueckenotte, L. (1992). *Pocket guide to geriatric assessment.* St. Louis: Mosby-Year Book.

Mathewson, Merrily K. (1991). *Pharmacotherapeutics: a nursing process approach.* Philadelphia: F.A. Davis.

North American Nursing Diagnosis Association. (1992). *Taxonomy revised with official nursing diagnoses.* St. Louis: 10th Conference.

Perry, A.G. and Potter, P.A. (1990). *Clinical nursing skills and techniques* (2nd ed.). St. Louis: Mosby-Year Book.

INDEX

ORDER FORM

Qty.	Title	Price	Total
	1995 Nurse's Trivia Calendar	$9.95	
	RN NCLEX Cards, 2nd ed.	$24.95	
	PN/VN Review Cards	$24.95	
	Nurse's Survival Guide, 2nd ed.	$24.95	
	The Body in Brief, 2nd ed.	$26.95	
	The OBRA Guideline for Quality Improvement in Long Term Care	$59.95	
	The OSHA Handbook	$79.95	
	Diagnostic & Laboratory Cards, 2nd ed.	$23.95	
	Drug Comparison Book, 2nd ed.	$29.95	
	The Skidmore-Roth Outline Series:		
	• Medical-Surgical Nursing	$18.95	
	• Pediatric Nursing	$16.95	
	• Obstetric Nursing	$16.95	
	Geriatric Long-Term Procedures & Treatments	$59.95	
	The RN NCLEX Series:		
	• Medical-Surgical Nursing	$18.95	
	• Pediatric Nursing	$18.95	
	• Obstetric Nursing	$18.95	
		Subtotal	
	Tax of 8.25% applies to Texas residents only.	8.25% Tax	
	UPS ground shipping $5 for first item, $1 each additional item.	Shipping	
		TOTAL	

Name	
Company	
Address	
City	State	Zip	Phone ( )

❏ Check enclosed   ❏ Visa   ❏ MasterCard   ❏ American Express

Credit Card Number

Card Holder Name

Signature   Expiration Date

To order call 1 (800) 825-3150 or fax us your order at (915) 877-4424

SKIDMORE-ROTH PUBLISHING, INC.
7730 Trade Center Avenue
El Paso, TX 79912